Carnivore Diet Air Fryer Cookbook for Beginners

2100 Days of Healthy and Delicious Recipes Easy-to-Make in Less Than 30 Minutes to Lose Weight, Stabilize Blood Sugar Levels and Increase Energy

John Labor

Warning – Disclaimer

The purpose of this book is to educate and entertain. The author or publisher does not guarantee that anyone following the techniques, suggestions, tips, ideas or strategies will have successful. The author and publisher shall have neither liability or responsibility to anyone with respect to any loss or damage caused or alleged to be caused, directly or indirectly, by the information contained in this book.

Bonus Guides

Are you ready to embark on a journey of culinary exploration and wellness empowerment? Get ready to unlock exclusive bonus guides that will revolutionize your cooking skills and empower you to embrace a healthier lifestyle.

In "**The Ultimate Air Fryer Starter Guidebook**", you'll unveil the secrets of air frying mastery. Say goodbye to greasy, calorie-laden dishes and hello to perfectly crispy, golden-brown creations. From succulent steaks to crispy pork belly, this comprehensive guide is filled with expert tips and step-by-step instructions to help you become an air frying virtuoso.

Ready to take charge of your health and embrace the carnivore lifestyle? Look no further than "**Embracing the Carnivore Way**". Dive into essential strategies for thriving on a meat-based diet while enjoying delicious and nutritious meals. From understanding the benefits of the carnivore diet to crafting balanced and flavorful dishes, this guide will equip you with the knowledge and tools to succeed with a carnivore lifestyle.

Plus, with "**Overcoming Obstacles: A Guide to Health on the Carnivore Diet**", you'll have a handy companion to navigate the potential challenges and health concerns of the carnivore diet with confidence. This guide offers solutions and strategies to help you maintain your health and well-being, ensuring you have the tools you need to overcome any hurdles you may encounter.

Don't miss out on these invaluable resources!

Scan the QR Code below to access your complimentary guides today. Whether you're a culinary enthusiast eager to expand your repertoire or an individual committed to optimizing your health with a carnivore diet, these guides are your key to a healthier and more flavorful life. Transform your cooking, transform your health – start scanning now!

Table of Contents

Introduction

Welcome to the "Carnivore Diet Air Fryer Cookbook for Beginners," your ultimate guide to transforming your meals and, by extension, your health, energy levels, and body. If you're reading this, chances are you're looking for a change. Maybe you're curious about the carnivore diet, intrigued by the simplicity it promises in a world cluttered with complex diet advice. Or perhaps you've heard about the health benefits and are eager to see if it can make a difference in your life. You might even be here because the idea of making delicious, nutritious meals in less than 30 minutes sounds too good to pass up. Whatever your reason, you're in the right place.

The carnivore diet, at its core, is about simplicity and returning to a way of eating that emphasizes whole, nutrient-dense animal foods. It's about cutting through the noise of dietary trends and focusing on what has sustained humans for millennia. But let's face it, adopting a new way of eating can be daunting, especially when it challenges conventional wisdom on nutrition and health. That's where this cookbook comes in. It's not just a collection of recipes; it's a roadmap to help you navigate this journey with ease and confidence.

One of the biggest hurdles for anyone adopting a new diet is the time and effort required to prepare meals. We live in a fast-paced world where time is a precious commodity. The thought of spending hours in the kitchen preparing meals can be a deal-breaker for many. This is where the magic of air frying and the carnivore diet come together beautifully. Air frying offers a way to prepare meals that are not only quick and easy but also healthier and packed with flavor. It's a game-changer for busy individuals who want to eat well without spending hours cooking.

But what about variety? One common misconception about the carnivore diet is that it's monotonous and restrictive. This couldn't be further from the truth, and this cookbook is proof of that. From succulent steaks and crispy bacon to tender fish and savory offal dishes, the recipes in this book showcase the incredible variety and culinary potential of animal-based foods. Whether you're a seasoned chef or a complete beginner, you'll find recipes here that will excite your taste buds and make mealtime something to look forward to.

Moreover, this cookbook is designed with your health and wellness goals in mind. Whether you're looking to lose weight, increase your energy levels, or simply improve your overall well-being, the carnivore diet has something to offer. The recipes in this book are crafted to provide maximum nutrition, helping you feel your best while enjoying delicious meals.

As you embark on this journey, remember that change doesn't happen overnight. It's a process, and there will be challenges along the way. But with this cookbook as your guide, you're well-equipped to face those challenges head-on. You'll learn not only how to prepare mouthwatering meals but also how to navigate the carnivore diet with confidence, making informed choices that align with your health and wellness goals.

So, let's get started. Open your mind, ready your air fryer, and prepare to embark on a culinary adventure that promises to transform the way you think about food, health, and cooking. Welcome to the carnivore diet air fryer revolution.

What is the Carnivore Diet?

The carnivore diet is a dietary plan that focuses exclusively on animal products, eschewing all forms of plant-based foods. It's a regimen that prioritizes meat, fish, eggs, and dairy products while eliminating fruits, vegetables, nuts, grains, and legumes. This approach to eating is rooted in the belief that human beings thrive on a meat-centric diet, drawing on historical precedents of hunter-gatherer societies as well as contemporary anecdotal evidence suggesting various health benefits.

At its heart, the carnivore diet is about simplicity and purity in nutrition. By consuming only animal products, adherents aim to reduce inflammation, cut out potential allergens and irritants found in many plant foods, and focus on nutrient-dense sources of protein and fat. This diet is rich in vitamins and minerals that are bioavailable—meaning the body can absorb and use them more efficiently—such as Vitamin B12, iron, zinc, and Omega-3 fatty acids, all crucial for maintaining health and vitality.

For those new to the concept, the idea of excluding all plant foods might seem daunting or even extreme. However, it's important to understand the rationale behind this choice. Proponents argue that many modern ailments stem from the agricultural revolution and the subsequent shift in human diets away from primarily animal-based foods. They suggest that by returning to a diet that more closely resembles that of our ancestors, individuals can alleviate some of these health issues, such as autoimmune diseases, digestive problems, and weight gain.

The carnivore diet also challenges conventional dietary wisdom that emphasizes the importance of fruits and vegetables for fiber and vitamins. Instead, it posits that animal products alone can provide all the necessary nutrients for optimal health, without the need for dietary supplements or fortified foods. This perspective encourages a reevaluation of current dietary guidelines and promotes further research into nutritional science.

For those embarking on this dietary journey, it's crucial to focus on variety and quality within the allowed foods. This means choosing grass-fed beef, pasture-raised poultry, wild-caught fish, and organic eggs, when possible, to maximize the nutritional benefits and minimize exposure to antibiotics, hormones, and pesticides. It also involves experimenting with different cuts of meat and types of animal products to ensure a broad intake of nutrients and to keep meals interesting and enjoyable.

Adopting the carnivore diet can be a significant lifestyle change, especially for individuals accustomed to a diet rich in plant-based foods. However, many find that the transition brings about positive changes in their health, energy levels, and overall well-being. It's a journey of discovery, learning how one's body responds to a meat-focused diet, and adjusting accordingly to meet personal health goals and dietary preferences. As with any dietary change, it's advisable to conduct thorough research, consult healthcare professionals, and listen to one's body to navigate this path safely and effectively.

Benefits of the carnivore diet

The carnivore diet, with its focus on consuming animal products, offers a myriad of health benefits that align perfectly with the goals of individuals seeking to improve their well-being, lose weight, and boost their energy levels. This diet simplifies nutrition by eliminating the guesswork involved in balancing a myriad of food groups, making it an appealing option for those with a busy lifestyle and a keen interest in maintaining an active, health-conscious life.

One of the most immediate benefits observed by many adopting this diet is weight loss. By focusing on high-protein and high-fat foods, the carnivore diet naturally leads to a reduction in appetite and an increase in satiety after meals. This can result in a lower caloric intake without the need for counting calories or feeling hungry, making weight loss both achievable and sustainable. The high protein content also supports muscle maintenance and growth, particularly beneficial for those engaged in regular physical activity.

Another significant advantage is the potential for improved digestion. Many people find that removing plant-based foods, which can contain irritants and anti-nutrients such as lectins, gluten, and fiber, leads to a reduction in bloating, gas, and other digestive issues. This can be particularly life-changing for individuals with sensitive digestive systems or conditions like irritable bowel syndrome (IBS).

The diet's emphasis on animal products also ensures a high intake of many essential nutrients that are more readily absorbed from animal sources. These include vitamins B12 and D, heme-iron, zinc, and omega-3 fatty acids, all crucial for maintaining optimal health. The bioavailability of these nutrients in animal products means the body can more efficiently utilize them, potentially leading to improved overall nutritional status and health outcomes.

Energy levels often see a marked improvement on the carnivore diet. This can be attributed to the stable blood sugar levels achieved by consuming a diet low in carbohydrates. Without the regular spikes and crashes associated with high-carb diets, individuals often report feeling more energized and alert throughout the day. This stable energy can support a more active lifestyle and improve mental clarity, making it easier to tackle daily tasks and engage in regular exercise.

Furthermore, the simplicity of the carnivore diet can be a significant time-saver, addressing one of the main pain points for many individuals: the time and effort required for meal preparation. With the focus on single-ingredient meals, cooking becomes less complicated and more efficient, freeing up time for other activities. This simplicity also makes it easier to stick to the diet, as the decision-making process around meals is streamlined, reducing the likelihood of falling back into less healthy eating habits.

Lastly, many adherents of the carnivore diet report improvements in skin health, mood, and overall well-being. While individual experiences vary, the reduction in sugar and processed foods, along with the increased intake of nutrient-dense animal products, may contribute to these positive effects. Clearer skin, better mood regulation, and a general feeling of well-being are often cited as compelling reasons to maintain this dietary lifestyle.

In summary, the carnivore diet offers a range of benefits that align with the goals of health-conscious individuals looking to lose weight, improve their nutritional intake, and lead a more active, fulfilling life. Its simplicity, combined with the potential for significant health improvements, makes it a compelling option for those seeking a straightforward approach to nutrition and well-being.

How to Combine Diabetic Diet and Air Frying

Combining the carnivore diet with air frying is a game-changer for anyone looking to streamline their meal prep while sticking to this health-focused lifestyle. Air frying offers a way to cook your carnivorous meals quickly, with minimal mess, and without sacrificing flavor or nutritional value. Here's how you can make the most of this dynamic duo to support your health goals, save time, and enjoy a variety of delicious, meat-based dishes.

First, understand the basics of air frying. An air fryer works by circulating hot air around the food, cooking it evenly and creating a crispy outer layer. This method requires little to no cooking oil, making it a healthier alternative to traditional frying. For the carnivore diet, this means you can enjoy the crispy texture of fried foods without straying from your dietary guidelines.

To get started, focus on selecting the right cuts of meat. Since the carnivore diet emphasizes animal products, opt for a variety of meats to keep your meals interesting. Beef, pork, chicken, fish, and lamb are all excellent choices. Consider cuts that will cook well in the air fryer, such as steaks, chops, wings, and fillets. The thickness of the meat can affect cooking time, so adjust accordingly.

Seasoning your meat is the next step. While the carnivore diet limits the use of plant-based seasonings, you can still achieve flavorful results with animal-based products. Salt is your best friend here, enhancing the natural flavors of the meat. For added variety, experiment with different types of salt, like Himalayan pink salt or smoked salt. You can also use animal fats to baste your meats before air frying, adding both flavor and moisture.

Now, let's talk about cooking times and temperatures. Each type of meat has its ideal cooking settings to ensure it's juicy and tender on the inside with a crispy exterior. Generally, you'll want to air fry steaks and chops at a higher temperature for a shorter time to achieve a perfect sear. Poultry and fish may require lower temperatures and longer cooking times. Always use a meat thermometer to ensure your meat reaches the safe internal temperature recommended for each type.

Incorporating variety into your meals is crucial to keeping the carnivore diet exciting and sustainable. Use your air fryer to experiment with different meats and cuts. Try air-fried bacon for a crispy treat, or make a batch of chicken wings with a crunchy exterior. Even seafood, like salmon fillets or shrimp, turns out wonderfully in the air fryer. The key is to be creative and open to trying new things.

Finally, consider meal planning and prep. One of the great advantages of air frying is its convenience. You can cook a variety of meats in advance and have them ready to eat throughout the week. This is especially beneficial for those with busy schedules who still want to maintain a healthy carnivore diet. Batch cooking and storing your meats properly will ensure you always have a quick, nutritious meal on hand.

By following these tips, you'll find that combining the carnivore diet with air frying not only simplifies your meal prep but also opens up a whole new world of delicious, nutritious options. Embrace the convenience and health benefits of this powerful combination to support your weight loss goals, increase your energy, and improve your overall well-being.

How to Use This Cookbook

Inside this cookbook, you'll find a variety of recipes meticulously crafted to meet the needs of a carnivore diet without compromising on flavor or satisfaction. From hearty breakfasts to satisfying main courses and savory snacks, each recipe is designed to maximize taste and nutritional value while being easy to prepare. The recipes are structured to help you make the most out of your air fryer, ensuring that you can enjoy a diverse array of meals with minimal prep and cleanup time.

This cookbook aims to:

- **Simplify Your Cooking**: With straightforward instructions and easy-to-find ingredients, preparing your meals will be a breeze.
- **Enhance Your Diet**: Each recipe is crafted to support your carnivore lifestyle, focusing on high-quality animal products that provide essential nutrients.
- **Save You Time**: By using an air fryer, you can cook meals quickly without sacrificing flavor or texture.
- **Inspire Creativity**: Discover new ways to prepare your favorite meats and explore different flavors and textures.

Recipe Categories

The "Carnivore Diet Air Fryer Cookbook for Beginners" is thoughtfully organized into several recipe categories to help you easily find and prepare meals that align with your dietary goals. Each category offers a variety of dishes that emphasize different types of meat to ensure you can enjoy a diverse and satisfying carnivore diet. The number one rule guiding these recipes is "eat healthy and eat varied." Here's how the recipes are categorized and the logic behind their creation:

- **Breakfast Recipes**: Start your day with hearty and nutritious breakfast options designed to fuel you through the morning. From crispy bacon strips to savory sausage patties and protein-packed egg muffins, these recipes ensure you begin your day with delicious and satisfying meals.

- **Pork Recipes**: Pork is a versatile and flavorful meat that can be prepared in numerous ways. This category includes a variety of pork-based dishes, such as tender pork belly bites, succulent pork chops, and flavorful ground pork patties, ensuring you never run out of delicious options.

- **Poultry Recipes**: Poultry is a staple in many diets due to its lean protein and versatility. Enjoy a range of chicken and turkey dishes, from crispy chicken wings to juicy turkey breast, each cooked to perfection in the air fryer. These recipes provide a great way to incorporate poultry into your carnivore diet.

- **Beef Recipes**: Beef lovers will find plenty to enjoy in this category, featuring a variety of cuts and preparations. From juicy ribeye steaks to flavorful ground beef patties and tender beef ribs, these recipes highlight the rich taste and texture of beef, making it a star of your meals.

- **Lamb Recipes**: Lamb offers a unique and rich flavor profile, perfect for those looking to diversify their meat intake. This category includes recipes for lamb chops, lamb burgers, and more, providing a range of options to enjoy this delectable meat.

- **Seafood and Fish Recipes**: Seafood and fish are excellent sources of lean protein and essential nutrients. This category offers recipes for salmon fillets, tuna steaks, and air-fried shrimp, among others. These dishes are perfect for adding variety to your carnivore diet while benefiting from the health advantages of seafood.

- **Game and Offal Recipes**: Game meats and offal are nutrient-dense options that can add an exciting twist to your meals. Explore recipes featuring venison, bison, duck liver, and more. These dishes are perfect for adventurous eaters looking to try something new and nutrient-packed.

- **Meaty Bowls and Wraps Recipes**: For those transitioning into the carnivore diet, this category offers recipes that incorporate small amounts of vegetables. These bowls and wraps provide a bridge between a traditional diet and a fully carnivorous one, making it easier to adapt. They are also great for serving guests who might not follow the carnivore diet, ensuring everyone enjoys a delicious meal.

- **Snacks and Sides Recipes**: Find a variety of snacks and side dishes to complement your main meals. From crispy pork rinds to mozzarella-stuffed chicken breasts, these recipes are perfect for satisfying cravings between meals or adding a little extra to your plate.

- **Homemade Sauces, Dips, and Seasonings Recipes**: Enhance the flavor of your dishes with homemade sauces, dips, and seasonings. These recipes ensure you can enjoy a variety of tastes and textures while staying true to the carnivore diet. From simple garlic butter to spicy dipping sauces, these additions will make your meals even more enjoyable.

Each recipe in this cookbook is crafted with a focus on foods suitable for the carnivore diet, primarily meat, fish, dairy products, and eggs. To ensure variety, different meats and cuts of meat are featured, along with various toppings and seasonings such as salt, pepper, onion, garlic, and other spices used in small quantities. This approach ensures that the diet remains enjoyable and sustainable, allowing you to reap the benefits without feeling restricted.

Whether you're a beginner or an expert in the carnivore diet, this cookbook provides the tools and inspiration needed to maintain a healthy and varied diet, all while using the convenience of an air fryer.

Scope and Variety

The "Carnivore Diet Air Fryer Cookbook for Beginners" offers an expansive collection of over 100 recipes, ensuring your meals are never monotonous. This extensive recipe collection covers everything from hearty breakfasts and succulent main dishes to satisfying snacks, providing endless options for every meal of the day.

With such a broad scope, this cookbook ensures long-term usability. The diverse array of recipes allows you to enjoy more than 2100 days of unique carnivorous meals without repetition. This variety helps you stay motivated and enthusiastic about your diet, making it easier to maintain over time. Whether you're new to the carnivore diet or a veteran pro, this cookbook is your key to a rich, varied, and satisfying dietary journey.

Efficiency and Convenience

Understanding the value of your time, I've meticulously crafted each recipe in this cookbook to be ready in 30 minutes or less. Whether you're juggling a hectic schedule during the week or enjoying a leisurely weekend, these recipes are designed to respect your precious time.

Delve into the world of carnivore cooking without sacrificing hours in the kitchen. With swift and convenient options available, you can delight in the flavors of your diet without the burden of lengthy cooking times. Embrace efficient cooking and turn every meal into a seamless experience with this indispensable cookbook.

A Little Disclaimer

In creating the "Carnivore Diet Air Fryer Cookbook for Beginners," I've chosen not to include images alongside the recipes. Why? Because conventional cookbook visuals often fail to capture the true essence of the culinary creations within.

Instead, I've curated an immersive visual experience to enrich your cooking journey. Introducing a companion compendium featuring breathtaking 4K color photos of every recipe in this book.

With these high-definition images, you'll witness the tantalizing textures and vibrant colors of each dish, from perfectly air-fried meats to mouthwatering sides. It's like having a culinary guide right beside you, enhancing your cooking endeavors and igniting your creativity.

To access this visual companion, simply **scan the QR Code** provided at the beginning of the book and follow the steps shown to you. It's that simple!

Furthermore, as a special bonus, you'll receive three exclusive guides:

Bonus 1: The Ultimate Air Fryer Starter Guidebook

Dive into the realm of air frying with expert tips and recipes to revolutionize your cooking. From crispy appetizers to succulent mains, this guidebook equips you with essential techniques and mouthwatering recipes to master the art of air frying.

Bonus 2: Embracing the Carnivore Way

Embark on a transformative journey toward a healthier lifestyle with my comprehensive handbook on the carnivore diet. Learn how to navigate the ins and outs of adopting and thriving on this meat-based diet, from meal planning and grocery shopping to sustainable habits and delicious recipes.

Bonus 3: Overcoming Obstacles

Navigate the potential challenges and health concerns of the carnivore diet with confidence. This guide offers solutions and strategies to help you maintain your health and well-being, ensuring you have the tools you need to overcome any hurdles you may encounter.

Breakfast Recipes

1. Air-Fried Bacon Strips

Preparation time: 5 minutes   **Cooking time:** 10 minutes   **Servings:** 2

Ingredients:

- 8 slices of thick-cut bacon

Directions:

1. Preheat your air fryer to 400°F (200°C). If your air fryer requires preheating, ensure it reaches the desired temperature before adding the bacon.
2. Arrange the bacon slices in a single layer in the air fryer basket. If your basket is small, you may need to cook them in batches to avoid overcrowding.
3. Cook for 10 minutes or until the bacon reaches the level of crispiness you desire. To ensure even cooking of the bacon, turn the slices halfway through cooking.
4. Once cooked, carefully remove the bacon strips from the air fryer basket and place them on a plate lined with paper towels to absorb any excess grease.
5. Serve immediately for the best texture and flavor.

Per serving: Calories: 315 kcal; Carbs: 0g; Fiber: 0g; Sugars: 0g; Protein: 21g; Saturated fat: 10g; Unsaturated fat: 5g.

2. Sausage Patties

Preparation time: 10 minutes   **Cooking time:** 15 minutes   **Servings:** 4

Ingredients:

- 1 pound ground pork
- 1 teaspoon salt
- 1/2 teaspoon ground black pepper
- 1 teaspoon sage
- 1 teaspoon thyme
- 1/2 teaspoon garlic powder
- 1/2 teaspoon onion powder
- 1/4 teaspoon cayenne pepper (optional for a spicy kick)

Directions:

1. In a large mixing bowl, combine the ground pork with salt, black pepper, sage, thyme, garlic powder, onion powder, and cayenne pepper (if using). Mix well until all the spices are evenly distributed throughout the meat.

2. Divide the mixture into eight equal portions. Roll each portion into a ball and then flatten into a patty shape, about 1/2 inch thick.

3. Preheat the air fryer to 400°F (200°C). If your air fryer requires preheating, make sure to do so before cooking.

4. Place the sausage patties in the air fryer basket in a single layer, ensuring they are not touching. You may need to cook them in batches depending on the size of your air fryer.

5. Cook for 15 minutes, flipping the patties halfway through the cooking time, until they are evenly browned and cooked through.

6. Remove the patties from the air fryer and let them rest for a couple of minutes before serving.

Per serving (= 2 patties): Calories: 339kcal; Carbs: 1g; Fiber: 0g; Sugars: 0g; Protein: 22g; Saturated fat: 12g; Unsaturated fat: 7g.

3. Egg Muffins

Preparation time: 10 minutes **Cooking time:** 15 minutes **Servings:** 2

Ingredients:

- 8 large eggs
- 1/2 cup of diced cooked bacon
- 1/4 cup of shredded cheddar cheese
- Salt and pepper to taste
- Cooking spray for greasing

Directions:

1. Preheat your air fryer to 300°F (150°C).
2. In a large bowl, whisk the eggs until well beaten. Season with salt and pepper.
3. Stir in the diced cooked bacon and shredded cheddar cheese into the egg mixture.
4. Grease a muffin tin that fits your air fryer basket with cooking spray.
5. Pour the egg mixture evenly into the muffin cups, filling each about two-thirds full.
6. Carefully place the muffin tin in the air fryer basket.
7. Cook for 15 minutes, or until the egg muffins are set and lightly golden on top.
8. Remove the muffin tin from the air fryer and let it cool for a couple of minutes before removing the egg muffins.
9. Serve warm and enjoy!

Per serving: Calories: 140kcal; Carbs: 1g; Fiber: 0g; Sugars: 1g; Protein: 12g; Saturated fat: 3.5g; Unsaturated fat: 2g.

4. Pork Belly Bites

Preparation time: 10 minutes **Cooking time:** 20 minutes **Servings:** 4

Ingredients:

- 1 pound pork belly, cut into 1-inch cubes
- 1 teaspoon salt
- 1 teaspoon black pepper
- 1 teaspoon garlic powder

Directions:

1. Preheat your air fryer to 400°F (200°C).
2. In a large bowl, toss the pork belly cubes with salt, pepper, and garlic powder until evenly coated.
3. Place the pork belly cubes in the air fryer basket in a single layer, ensuring they are not overcrowded to allow for even cooking.
4. Cook for 10 minutes, then shake the basket or use tongs to flip the pork belly bites.
5. Continue cooking for an additional 10 minutes or until the pork belly bites are golden brown and crispy to your liking.
6. Remove the pork belly bites from the air fryer.
7. Before serving, let the pork belly bites rest for a few minutes.

Per serving: Calories: 507kcal; Carbs: 0g; Fiber: 0g; Sugars: 0g; Protein: 11g; Saturated fat: 18g; Unsaturated fat: 13g.

5. Steak & Eggs

Preparation time: 5 minutes **Cooking time:** 20 minutes **Servings:** 2

Ingredients:

- 2 ribeye steaks (about 1-inch thick)
- 4 large eggs
- Salt and pepper, to taste
- 1 tablespoon of olive oil (for greasing)

Directions:

1. Preheat your air fryer to 400°F (200°C). Lightly grease the air fryer basket with olive oil.
2. Season the ribeye steaks generously with salt and pepper on both sides.
3. Place the steaks in the air fryer basket and cook for 10 minutes for medium-rare, or adjust the time according to your preferred level of doneness. Flip the steaks halfway through the cooking time.
4. Once the steaks are cooked to your liking, transfer them to a plate and let them rest for a few minutes. This helps the juices redistribute, making your steak juicier.

5. While the steaks are resting, crack the eggs into the air fryer basket. You might want to use an air fryer accessory or a heat-resistant ramekin to hold the eggs if you prefer them in a specific shape.

6. Cook the eggs for 3-5 minutes at 370°F (187°C) or until they reach your desired level of doneness.

7. Serve the steaks with the fried eggs on top or on the side, depending on your preference.

Per serving: Calories: 622kcal; Carbs: 1g; Fiber: 0g; Sugars: 0g; Protein: 52g; Saturated fat: 18g; Unsaturated fat: 25g.

6. Chicken Liver Pâté

Preparation time: 10 minutes   **Cooking time:** 15 minutes   **Servings:** 4

Ingredients:

- 1 pound chicken livers, cleaned and trimmed
- 2 tablespoons unsalted butter
- 1/4 cup heavy cream
- 1 small onion, finely chopped
- 2 cloves garlic, minced

- 1 teaspoon fresh thyme leaves
- 1/2 teaspoon salt
- 1/4 teaspoon black pepper
- 2 tablespoons brandy or cognac (optional)

Directions:

1. Preheat the air fryer to 370°F.

2. In a skillet over medium heat, melt 1 tablespoon of butter. Add the onion and garlic, sautéing until translucent, about 3-4 minutes.

3. Add the chicken livers to the skillet, cooking until they are browned on the outside but still slightly pink in the middle, approximately 5 minutes.

4. Stir in the thyme, salt, pepper, and brandy (if using), cooking for an additional 2 minutes.

5. Transfer the liver mixture to a food processor, adding the remaining butter and heavy cream. Blend until the mixture is smooth.

6. Spoon the pâté into a serving dish or individual ramekins. For best flavor, cover and refrigerate for at least 2 hours before serving.

7. Serve chilled. The pâté can be stored in the refrigerator for up to 5 days.

Per serving: Calories: 292kcal; Carbs: 4g; Fiber: 0g; Sugars: 1g; Protein: 19g; Saturated fat: 10g; Unsaturated fat: 5g.

7. Lamb Chops

Preparation time: 5 minutes   **Cooking time:** 12 minutes   **Servings:** 2

Ingredients:

- 4 lamb chops, about 1 inch thick
- 1 tablespoon olive oil
- 1 teaspoon salt
- 1/2 teaspoon black pepper
- 1/2 teaspoon rosemary, dried
- 1/2 teaspoon garlic powder

Directions:

1. Preheat your air fryer to 400°F (200°C).
2. Rub each lamb chop with olive oil. In a small bowl, mix together salt, pepper, rosemary, and garlic powder. Sprinkle the seasoning mix evenly over both sides of the lamb chops.
3. Place the lamb chops in the air fryer basket, ensuring they are not touching to allow for even cooking.
4. Cook for 6 minutes, then flip the lamb chops over and cook for an additional 6 minutes for medium-rare or adjust the time according to your preferred level of doneness.
5. Once cooked, let the lamb chops rest for 3 minutes before serving to allow the juices to redistribute.

Per serving: Calories: 310kcal; Carbs: 0g; Fiber: 0g; Sugars: 0g; Protein: 25g; Saturated fat: 7g; Unsaturated fat: 5g.

8. Salmon Fillets

Preparation time: 5 minutes   **Cooking time:** 10 minutes   **Servings:** 2

Ingredients:

- 2 salmon fillets (6 ounces each)
- 1 tablespoon olive oil
- Salt and pepper to taste
- Optional: Lemon wedges and fresh dill for garnish

Directions:

1. Preheat your air fryer to 400°F (200°C).
2. Pat the salmon fillets dry with paper towels. This step is crucial for getting that perfect crispy exterior.
3. Rub each fillet with olive oil, then season generously with salt and pepper. If you're feeling adventurous, a sprinkle of your favorite herbs can add an extra layer of flavor.
4. Place the salmon fillets in the air fryer basket, skin-side down. Ensure they are not touching to allow for even cooking.

5. Cook for 10 minutes, or until the salmon easily flakes with a fork. There's no need to flip the fillets halfway through.

6. Once done, carefully remove the salmon from the air fryer and let it rest for a couple of minutes. This rest period lets the juices redistribute, ensuring your salmon is moist and flavorful.

7. Serve immediately, garnished with lemon wedges and fresh dill if desired.

Per serving: Calories: 280kcal; Carbs: 0g; Fiber: 0g; Sugars: 0g; Protein: 34g; Saturated fat: 4g; Unsaturated fat: 10g.

9. Turkey Bacon Crisp

Preparation time: 5 minutes   **Cooking time:** 10 minutes   **Servings:** 4

Ingredients:

- 8 slices of turkey bacon

Directions:

1. Preheat your air fryer to 360°F (182°C).

2. Arrange the turkey bacon slices in a single layer in the air fryer basket. You may need to work in batches depending on the size of your air fryer.

3. Cook for 10 minutes, flipping the bacon slices halfway through the cooking time, until they reach your desired level of crispiness.

4. Once cooked, carefully remove the turkey bacon from the air fryer and place them on a paper towel-lined plate to absorb any excess fat.

5. Serve immediately for the best texture and flavor.

Per serving: Calories: 70kcal; Carbs: 0g; Fiber: 0g; Sugars: 0g; Protein: 6g; Saturated fat: 2g; Unsaturated fat: 1g.

10. Duck Breast

Preparation time: 5 minutes   **Cooking time:** 20 minutes   **Servings:** 2

Ingredients:

- 2 duck breasts (about 6 ounces each)
- Salt, to taste
- Freshly ground black pepper, to taste

Directions:

1. Preheat your air fryer to 360°F (182°C).

2. Score the skin of the duck breasts in a diamond pattern, being careful not to cut into the meat. This helps render the fat and makes the skin crispy.

3. Season both sides of the duck breasts with salt and pepper.

4. Place the duck breasts skin-side down in the air fryer basket.

5. Cook for 10 minutes, then flip the duck breasts over and cook for an additional 10 minutes, or until the internal temperature reaches 135°F (57°C) for medium-rare.

6. Remove the duck breasts from the air fryer and let them rest for 5 minutes. The resting time allows the juices to redistribute, ensuring a moist and flavorful meat.

7. Slice and serve immediately.

Per serving: Calories: 340kcal; Carbs: 0g; Fiber: 0g; Sugars: 0g; Protein: 45g; Saturated fat: 6g; Unsaturated fat: 5g.

11. Venison Sausage

Preparation time: 15 minutes   **Cooking time:** 10 minutes   **Servings:** 4

Ingredients:

- 1 pound ground venison
- 1 teaspoon salt
- 1/2 teaspoon black pepper
- 1 teaspoon garlic powder
- 1 teaspoon onion powder

- 1/2 teaspoon dried thyme
- 1/2 teaspoon smoked paprika
- 1/4 teaspoon cayenne pepper (optional for a spicy kick)
- 2 tablespoon cold water

Directions:

1. In a large mixing bowl, combine the ground venison with salt, black pepper, garlic powder, onion powder, dried thyme, smoked paprika, and cayenne pepper (if using). Mix well to ensure the spices are evenly distributed throughout the meat.

2. Gradually add the cold water to the venison mixture. This helps to keep the sausage moist during cooking. Mix until well combined.

3. Divide the mixture into equal portions and shape each portion into a sausage link or patty, depending on your preference.

4. Preheat your air fryer to 400°F (200°C). Once heated, place the venison sausages in the air fryer basket, ensuring they are not touching to allow for even cooking.

5. Cook for 10 minutes, turning the sausages halfway through the cooking time, until they are browned and cooked through.

6. Carefully remove the sausages from the air fryer and let them rest for a couple of minutes before serving.

Per serving: Calories: 160kcal; Carbs: 1g; Fiber: 0g; Sugars: 0g; Protein: 22g; Saturated fat: 2g; Unsaturated fat: 1g.

12. Bison Burger

Preparation time: 10 minutes **Cooking time:** 15 minutes **Servings:** 2

Ingredients:

- 1 pound ground bison meat
- 1 teaspoon salt
- 1/2 teaspoon black pepper
- 1/2 teaspoon garlic powder
- 1/2 teaspoon onion powder
- Optional: 2 slices of cheese (for topping)

Directions:

1. Preheat your air fryer to 375°F (190°C).
2. In a bowl, mix the ground bison meat with salt, pepper, garlic powder, and onion powder until well combined.
3. Divide the mixture into two equal portions and shape each into a burger patty.
4. Place the patties in the air fryer basket, ensuring they are not touching to allow for even cooking.
5. Cook for about 15 minutes, flipping halfway through, or until the internal temperature reaches 160°F (71°C) for a well-done burger. If you're adding cheese, place it on top of the patties during the last 2 minutes of cooking.
6. Once cooked, remove the burgers from the air fryer and let them rest for a couple of minutes before serving.

Per serving: Calories: 280kcal; Carbs: 0g; Fiber: 0g; Sugars: 0g; Protein: 40g; Saturated fat: 8g; Unsaturated fat: 4g.

Pork Recipes

13. Pork Belly Crisp

Preparation time: 5 minutes   **Cooking time:** 25 minutes   **Servings:** 4

Ingredients:

- 1 pound pork belly, skin-on
- 1 teaspoon salt
- 1/2 teaspoon black pepper

Directions:

1. Start by scoring the skin of the pork belly in a diamond pattern, ensuring not to cut too deep into the fat.
2. Rub the salt and pepper evenly over the skin and into the scores you've made. This not only seasons the meat but helps the skin to crisp up beautifully.
3. Preheat your air fryer to 400°F (200°C). If your air fryer recommends preheating, ensure it's at the right temperature before cooking.
4. Place the pork belly in the air fryer basket, skin-side up. Make sure it's placed in a single layer for even cooking.
5. Cook for 25 minutes, or until the skin is puffed and crisp to the touch. The exact time may vary depending on the thickness of the pork belly and your air fryer model.
6. Once done, remove the pork belly from the air fryer and let it rest for a few minutes. This allows the juices to redistribute, making every bite as delicious as the next.
7. Slice into bite-sized pieces and serve immediately for the best texture and flavor.

Per serving: Calories: 560kcal; Carbs: 0g; Fiber: 0g; Sugars: 0g; Protein: 11g; Saturated fat: 20g; Unsaturated fat: 25g.

14. Asian-Inspired Pork Meatballs

Preparation time: 10 minutes   **Cooking time:** 15 minutes   **Servings:** 4

Ingredients:

- 1 pound ground pork
- 2 onions, finely chopped
- 2 cloves garlic, minced
- 1 tablespoon soy sauce (or tamari for gluten-free)
- 1 teaspoon grated ginger
- Salt and pepper, to taste

For the Sauce:

- 1/4 cup soy sauce (or tamari for gluten-free)
- 1 tablespoon honey
- 1 teaspoon grated ginger
- 1 clove garlic, minced

Directions:

1. 1. In a large mixing bowl, combine the ground pork, onions, minced garlic, soy sauce, grated ginger, salt, and pepper. Mix until well combined.
2. 2. Preheat the air fryer to 375°F (190°C).
3. 3. Shape the pork mixture into small meatballs, about 1 inch in diameter, and place them on a greased air fryer basket or tray, leaving space between each meatball.
4. 4. Cook the meatballs in the air fryer for 15 minutes, shaking the basket or turning the meatballs halfway through cooking, until they are browned and cooked through.
5. 5. While the meatballs are cooking, prepare the sauce. In a small saucepan, combine the soy sauce, honey, grated ginger, and minced garlic. Cook over medium heat for 2-3 minutes, stirring occasionally, until the sauce has thickened slightly.
6. 6. Once the meatballs are cooked, transfer them to a serving dish and drizzle the sauce over the top.

Per serving: Calories: 290kcal; Carbs: 4g; Fiber: 1g; Sugars: 2g; Protein: 17g; Fat: 21g; Saturated fat: 6g; Unsaturated fat: 15g

15. Pork Loin Roast

Preparation time: 10 minutes   **Cooking time:** 20 minutes   **Servings:** 4

Ingredients:

- 2 pound pork loin roast
- 1 teaspoon salt
- 1/2 teaspoon black pepper
- 1 teaspoon garlic powder
- 1/2 teaspoon onion powder (optional)
- 1 tablespoon olive oil

Directions:

1. Start by preheating your air fryer to 390°F (200°C).
2. While the air fryer is heating, pat the pork loin dry with paper towels. This will help to achieve a crispy exterior.
3. Rub the entire surface of the pork loin with olive oil, then season evenly with salt, pepper, garlic powder, and onion powder, if using.
4. Place the seasoned pork loin in the air fryer basket.
5. Cook for 20 minutes, or until the internal temperature of the pork loin reaches 145°F (63°C) when checked with a meat thermometer.

6. Once cooked, remove the pork loin from the air fryer and let it rest for 5 minutes before slicing. Resting allows the juices to redistribute throughout the meat, ensuring it's moist and flavorful.

7. Slice the pork loin roast into thick or thin slices, according to your preference, and serve immediately.

Per serving: Calories: 238kcal; Carbs: 0g; Fiber: 0g; Sugars: 0g; Protein: 35g; Saturated fat: 5g; Unsaturated fat: 8g.

16. Chorizo Bites

Preparation time: 5 minutes   **Cooking time:** 10 minutes   **Servings:** 4

Ingredients:

- 1 pound chorizo sausage, casing removed
- Optional: 1/4 teaspoon chili powder for extra heat

Directions:

1. Preheat your air fryer to 400°F (200°C).

2. If using, mix the chorizo with the chili powder in a bowl to evenly distribute the extra heat throughout the sausage.

3. Form the chorizo into small, bite-sized balls, about 1 inch in diameter. This should yield approximately 16 chorizo bites.

4. Place the chorizo bites in the air fryer basket in a single layer, ensuring they are not touching to allow for even cooking. You may need to cook them in batches depending on the size of your air fryer.

5. Cook for 10 minutes, or until the chorizo bites are fully cooked and have a crispy exterior. Halfway through the cooking time, shake the basket or use tongs to turn the bites for even cooking.

6. Carefully remove the chorizo bites from the air fryer and let them rest for a couple of minutes before serving.

Per serving: Calories: 298kcal; Carbs: 1g; Fiber: 0g; Sugars: 0g; Protein: 21g; Saturated fat: 13g; Unsaturated fat: 7g.

17. Spare Ribs

Preparation time: 10 minutes   **Cooking time:** 20 minutes   **Servings:** 4

Ingredients:

- 2 pounds pork spare ribs
- 1 tablespoon salt
- 1 teaspoon black pepper
- 1 teaspoon garlic powder

Directions:

1. Preheat your air fryer to 380°F (193°C).
2. Pat the spare ribs dry with paper towels to ensure proper seasoning adhesion and to help achieve a crispy texture.
3. In a small bowl, mix the salt, black pepper, and garlic powder (if using). Rub this seasoning mix all over the spare ribs, ensuring even coverage.
4. Place the seasoned spare ribs in the air fryer basket. Depending on the size of your air fryer, you may need to cut the ribs into smaller sections to fit.
5. Cook for 20 minutes, flipping the ribs halfway through the cooking time to ensure they are evenly cooked and crisped on all sides.
6. Once the ribs are cooked through and have reached an internal temperature of 145°F (63°C), remove them from the air fryer and let them rest for a few minutes. This resting period allows the juices to redistribute, making the ribs even more tender and flavorful.
7. Serve hot and enjoy the succulent taste of air-fried spare ribs.

Per serving: Calories: 498kcal; Carbs: 0g; Fiber: 0g; Sugars: 0g; Protein: 24g; Saturated fat: 20g; Unsaturated fat: 22g.

18. Ham Steaks

Preparation time: 5 minutes   **Cooking time:** 10 minutes   **Servings:** 2

Ingredients:

- 2 ham steaks (about 1/2 inch thick)
- 1 teaspoon black pepper
- 1 tablespoon water (to help create a moist cooking environment in the air fryer)

Directions:

1. Preheat your air fryer to 380°F (193°C).
2. Pat the ham steaks dry with paper towels to remove any excess moisture. This step helps to achieve a slightly crispy edge.
3. Season both sides of the ham steaks with black pepper.
4. Place the ham steaks in the air fryer basket. To prevent them from curling up as they cook, you can score the edges or place a small heat-proof object on top.
5. Add 1 tablespoon of water to the bottom of the air fryer basket. This helps to keep the ham moist during cooking.
6. Cook for 10 minutes, flipping the ham steaks halfway through the cooking time, until they are heated through and have a slightly crispy exterior.

7. Remove the ham steaks from the air fryer and let them rest for 2 minutes before serving. This allows the juices to redistribute, ensuring your ham steaks are moist and flavorful.

Per serving: Calories: 210kcal; Carbs: 0g; Fiber: 0g; Sugars: 0g; Protein: 30g; Saturated fat: 3g; Unsaturated fat: 3g.

19. Pork Chops

Preparation time: 5 minutes   **Cooking time:** 12 minutes   **Servings:** 2

Ingredients:

- 2 pork chops, about 1 inch thick
- 1 teaspoon salt
- 1/2 teaspoon black pepper
- 1/2 teaspoon garlic powder
- 1 tablespoon olive oil

Directions:

1. Preheat your air fryer to 400°F (200°C).
2. Rub both sides of the pork chops with olive oil. Season evenly with salt, pepper, and garlic powder (if using).
3. Place the pork chops in the air fryer basket, ensuring they do not overlap to allow for even cooking.
4. Cook for 6 minutes, then flip the pork chops over and cook for an additional 6 minutes, or until the internal temperature reaches 145°F (63°C) for a perfectly cooked chop.
5. Remove the pork chops from the air fryer and let them rest for 3 minutes before serving. This resting period allows the juices to redistribute throughout the meat, ensuring your chops are moist and flavorful.

Per serving: Calories: 310kcal; Carbs: 0g; Fiber: 0g; Sugars: 0g; Protein: 29g; Saturated fat: 5g; Unsaturated fat: 8g.

20. Bacon and Egg Bites

Preparation time: 10 minutes   **Cooking time:** 15 minutes   **Servings:** 4

Ingredients:

- 8 slices bacon
- 4 large eggs
- Salt and pepper, to taste
- Chopped fresh chives, for garnish (optional)

Directions:

1. Preheat the air fryer to 350°F.
2. Cut each bacon slice in half and line the wells of an air fryer basket with the bacon, forming a cup shape.
3. Crack an egg into each bacon cup.
4. Season using salt and pepper.
5. Air fry 15 minutes, or until the egg whites are set but then the yolks are still runny.
6. Garnish using chopped chives if desired.

Per serving: Calories: 195kcal; Carbs: 0g; Fiber: 0g; Sugars: 0g; Protein: 11g; Saturated fat: 5g; Unsaturated fat: 11g.

21. Sausage Links

Preparation time: 15 minutes   **Cooking time:** 10 minutes   **Servings:** 4

Ingredients:

- 1 pound ground pork
- 1 teaspoon sea salt
- 1/2 teaspoon black pepper
- 1 teaspoon dried sage
- 1/2 teaspoon dried thyme
- 1/4 teaspoon nutmeg

- 1/4 teaspoon cayenne pepper (optional for a spicy kick)
- Natural sausage casings, rinsed and prepared according to package instructions

Directions:

1. In a large mixing bowl, combine ground pork, sea salt, black pepper, dried sage, dried thyme, nutmeg, and cayenne pepper (if using). Mix thoroughly to ensure the spices are evenly distributed throughout the meat.
2. If using a sausage stuffer, attach the prepared casings to the stuffer's nozzle. Carefully feed the seasoned pork mixture into the stuffer and fill the casings, being careful not to overfill. Twist or tie off the sausages into 6-inch links.
3. Preheat the air fryer to 400°F (200°C).
4. Place the sausage links in the air fryer basket, ensuring they are not touching to allow for even cooking. You may need to cook them in batches depending on the size of your air fryer.
5. Cook for 10 minutes, turning the sausages halfway through the cooking time, until they are golden brown, and the internal temperature reaches 160°F (71°C).
6. Remove the sausage links from the air fryer and let them rest for a few minutes before serving.

Per serving (= 2 links): Calories: 290kcal; Carbs: 0g; Fiber: 0g; Sugars: 0g; Protein: 19g; Saturated fat: 10g; Unsaturated fat: 5g.

22. Ground Pork Patties

Preparation time: 10 minutes   **Cooking time:** 15 minutes   **Servings:** 4

Ingredients:

- 1 pound ground pork
- 1 teaspoon sea salt
- 1/2 teaspoon black pepper
- Optional: 1/2 teaspoon smoked paprika for a hint of smokiness

Directions:

1. In a large bowl, mix together the ground pork, sea salt, black pepper, and smoked paprika (if using) until well combined.
2. Divide the mixture into four equal parts. Roll each part into a ball and then flatten into a patty shape, about 3/4 inch thick.
3. Preheat the air fryer to 400°F (200°C). If your air fryer model requires preheating, ensure it's at the correct temperature before cooking.
4. Place the patties in the air fryer basket, making sure they are not touching to allow for even cooking. You may need to cook them in batches depending on the size of your air fryer.
5. Cook for 15 minutes, flipping the patties halfway through the cooking time, until they are golden brown and cooked through.
6. Remove the patties from the air fryer and let them rest for a few minutes on a plate before serving.

Per serving: Calories: 290kcal; Carbs: 0g; Fiber: 0g; Sugars: 0g; Protein: 20g; Saturated fat: 10g; Unsaturated fat: 9g.

23. Pork Tenderloin

Preparation time: 5 minutes   **Cooking time:** 20 minutes   **Servings:** 4

Ingredients:

- 1 pork tenderloin (about 1-1.5 pounds)
- 1 teaspoon salt
- 1/2 teaspoon black pepper
- 1/2 teaspoon garlic powder
- 1/2 teaspoon onion powder

Directions:

1. Start by preheating your air fryer to 400°F (200°C).
2. While the air fryer is heating, pat the pork tenderloin dry with paper towels. This will help achieve a better sear.
3. Season the tenderloin evenly with salt, pepper, garlic powder, and onion powder. Ensure the entire surface is covered for maximum flavor.

4. Place the seasoned pork tenderloin in the air fryer basket. Make sure it's positioned in the center for a better cooking.

5. Cook for 20 minutes, flipping the tenderloin halfway through the cooking time to ensure it cooks evenly on all sides.

6. Check the internal temperature of the pork tenderloin with a meat thermometer. The USDA recommends a minimum internal temperature of 145°F (63°C) for pork.

7. Once cooked, remove the pork tenderloin from the air fryer and let it rest for 3-5 minutes before slicing. Resting allows the juices to redistribute, making the meat more tender and flavorful.

8. Slice the tenderloin and serve immediately.

Per serving: Calories: 224kcal; Carbs: 0g; Fiber: 0g; Sugars: 0g; Protein: 30g; Saturated fat: 2g; Unsaturated fat: 3g

24. Carnivore Pork "Pizza"

Preparation time: 15 minutes   **Cooking time:** 15 minutes   **Servings:** 2

Ingredients:

- 1 pound ground pork
- 1 teaspoon salt
- 1/2 teaspoon black pepper
- 1/2 teaspoon garlic powder

- 1 cup shredded mozzarella cheese
- 5 slices of pepperoni (optional)
- 1/2 cup cooked bacon pieces

Directions:

1. In a bowl, mix the ground pork with salt, black pepper, and garlic powder until well combined.

2. Press the pork mixture into a thin layer on a parchment-lined air fryer basket, shaping it into a round pizza base.

3. Preheat the air fryer to 400°F (200°C).

4. Cook the pork base for 10 minutes, or until it starts to brown and crisp up on the edges.

5. Carefully remove the basket from the air fryer and sprinkle the cooked pork base with shredded mozzarella cheese, pepperoni slices (optional), and bacon pieces.

6. Return the basket to the air fryer and cook for an additional 5 minutes, or until the cheese is melted and bubbly.

7. Remove the Carnivore Pork Pizza from the air fryer and let it cool for a couple of minutes before slicing and serving.

Per serving: Calories: 720kcal; Carbs: 0g; Fiber: 0g; Sugars: 0g; Protein: 48g; Saturated fat: 27g; Unsaturated fat: 20g.

Poultry Recipes

25. Chicken Thighs

Preparation time: 5 minutes   **Cooking time:** 20 minutes   **Servings:** 4

Ingredients:

- 4 chicken thighs, bone-in and skin-on
- 1 teaspoon salt
- 1/2 teaspoon black pepper

Directions:

1. Preheat your air fryer to 390°F (200°C).
2. Pat the chicken thighs dry with paper towels to remove any excess moisture. This step is crucial for achieving crispy skin.
3. Season both sides of the chicken thighs evenly with salt and pepper.
4. Place the chicken thighs in the air fryer basket, skin-side up, ensuring they are not touching to allow for even cooking.
5. Cook for 20 minutes, or until the chicken skin is crispy and golden, and the internal temperature reaches 165°F (74°C) when checked with a meat thermometer.
6. Remove the chicken thighs from the air fryer and let them rest for a few minutes before serving. This allows the juices to redistribute, ensuring every bite is moist and flavorful.

Per serving: Calories: 210kcal; Carbs: 0g; Fiber: 0g; Sugars: 0g; Protein: 31g; Saturated fat: 4g; Unsaturated fat: 8g.

26. Turkey Meatballs

Preparation time: 15 minutes   **Cooking time:** 15 minutes   **Servings:** 4

Ingredients:

- 1 pound ground turkey
- 1 teaspoon salt
- 1/2 teaspoon black pepper
- 1/2 teaspoon garlic powder
- 1/2 teaspoon onion powder (optional)

Directions:

1. In a large bowl, combine the ground turkey, salt, black pepper, garlic powder, and onion powder. Mix until the ingredients are well incorporated.
2. Form the mixture into small balls, about 1 inch in diameter. This should yield approximately 16 meatballs.

3. Preheat your air fryer to 400°F (200°C).

4. Place the meatballs in the air fryer basket, ensuring they are not touching to allow for even cooking. You may need to cook them in batches depending on the size of your air fryer.

5. Cook for 15 minutes, or until the meatballs are golden brown on the outside and reach an internal temperature of 165°F (74°C).

6. Remove the meatballs from the air fryer and let them rest for a few minutes before serving.

Per serving: Calories: 170kcal; Carbs: 0g; Fiber: 0g; Sugars: 0g; Protein: 22g; Saturated fat: 3g; Unsaturated fat: 2g.

27. Spices-Stuffed Chicken

Preparation time: 15 minutes   **Cooking time:** 15 minutes   **Servings:** 4

Ingredients:

- 4 boneless skinless chicken breast
- 1 small, sliced onion
- 1/2 small sliced green pepper (optional)
- 1 tablespoon olive oil
- 1 teaspoon chili powder
- 1 teaspoon ground cumin
- 1 teaspoon minced cilantro
- 1/2 teaspoon salt
- 1/4 teaspoon garlic powder
- 4 slices cheddar cheese

Directions:

1. Preheat air fryer to 375°.

2. In the thickest part of each chicken breast, cut a pocket horizontally and fill with onion and green pepper.

3. In a small bowl, mix olive oil and seasonings; rub over chicken.

4. In batches, place chicken in air-fryer basket.

5. Cook 6 minutes.

6. Top chicken with cheese slices; secure with toothpicks.

7. Cook until a thermometer inserted in chicken reads at least 165°, 8 minutes longer.

8. Discard toothpicks and serve immediately.

Per serving: Calories: 347kcal; Carbs: 5g; Fiber: 1g; Sugar: 1g; Protein: 42g; Saturated Fat: 7g; Unsatured Fat: 10g.

28. Chicken Wings

Preparation time: 5 minutes   **Cooking time:** 20 minutes   **Servings:** 4

Ingredients:

- 2 pounds chicken wings, tips removed and wings cut into drumettes and flats
- 1 teaspoon salt
- 1/2 teaspoon black pepper
- Optional: Your favorite seasoning for extra flavor

Directions:

1. Preheat your air fryer to 400°F (200°C).
2. Pat the chicken wings dry with paper towels. This step is crucial for achieving crispy skin.
3. Season the wings evenly with salt and black pepper. If you're using additional seasonings, add them at this stage.
4. Arrange the wings in a single layer in the air fryer basket, ensuring they are not touching to allow for proper air circulation.
5. Cook for 20 minutes, flipping the wings halfway through the cooking time, until they are golden brown and crispy.
6. Once cooked, carefully remove the chicken wings from the air fryer and let them rest for a few minutes on a plate.
7. Serve hot and enjoy the deliciously crispy texture and rich flavor of your air-fried chicken wings.

Per serving: Calories: 210kcal; Carbs: 0g; Fiber: 0g; Sugars: 0g; Protein: 18g; Saturated fat: 6g; Unsaturated fat: 9g.

29. Turkey Breast

Preparation time: 5 minutes   **Cooking time:** 30 minutes   **Servings:** 4

Ingredients:

- 1 turkey breast (about 3 pounds), boneless and skin-on
- 1 teaspoon salt
- 1/2 teaspoon black pepper
- 1/2 teaspoon garlic powder

Directions:

1. Preheat your air fryer to 350°F (175°C).
2. Pat the turkey breast dry with paper towels. This will help the skin get extra crispy.
3. Season the turkey breast evenly with salt, pepper, and garlic powder (if using).
4. Place the turkey breast in the air fryer basket, skin-side up.

5. Cook for 45 minutes, or until the internal temperature reaches 165°F (74°C) when checked with a meat thermometer inserted into the thickest part of the breast.

6. Once cooked, carefully remove the turkey breast from the air fryer and let it rest for 10 minutes before slicing. Resting allows the juices to redistribute throughout the meat, ensuring it's moist and flavorful.

7. Slice the turkey breast and serve immediately.

Per serving: Calories: 214kcal; Carbs: 0g; Fiber: 0g; Sugars: 0g; Protein: 30g; Saturated fat: 1g; Unsaturated fat: 1g.

30. Chicken Drumsticks

Preparation time: 5 minutes   **Cooking time:** 20 minutes   **Servings:** 4

Ingredients:

- 8 chicken drumsticks
- 1 teaspoon salt
- 1/2 teaspoon black pepper
- 1/2 teaspoon garlic powder

Directions:

1. Preheat your air fryer to 400°F (200°C).
2. Pat the chicken drumsticks dry with paper towels to remove any excess moisture. This step is crucial for achieving crispy skin.
3. Season the drumsticks evenly with salt and black pepper. Add garlic powder if desired.
4. Place the seasoned drumsticks in the air fryer basket, ensuring they are not touching to allow for even cooking.
5. Cook for 20 minutes, turning the drumsticks halfway through the cooking time to ensure they are evenly crisped and golden brown.
6. Check the internal temperature with a meat thermometer. The USDA recommends a minimum internal temperature of 165°F (74°C) for chicken.
7. Remove the drumsticks from the air fryer and let them rest for a few minutes before serving. This allows the juices to redistribute, ensuring your drumsticks are moist and flavorful.

Per serving: Calories: 220kcal; Carbs: 0g; Fiber: 0g; Sugars: 0g; Protein: 24g; Saturated fat: 3g; Unsaturated fat: 4g.

31. Quail

Preparation time: 5 minutes   **Cooking time:** 15 minutes   **Servings:** 2

Ingredients:

- 4 whole quails, cleaned and patted dry
- 1 teaspoon salt
- 1/2 teaspoon black pepper
- 1/2 teaspoon smoked paprika

Directions:

1. Preheat your air fryer to 390°F (200°C).
2. Season the quails evenly with salt, pepper, and smoked paprika.
3. Place the quails in the air fryer basket, ensuring they are not touching to allow for even cooking.
4. Cook for 15 minutes, flipping halfway through the cooking time, until the quails are golden brown and the internal temperature reaches 165°F (74°C).
5. Remove the quails from the air fryer and let them rest for a few minutes before serving. This resting period allows the juices to redistribute, ensuring each bite is moist and flavorful.

Per serving: Calories: 310kcal; Carbs: 0g; Fiber: 0g; Sugars: 0g; Protein: 52g; Saturated fat: 8g; Unsaturated fat: 5g.

32. Chicken Liver

Preparation time: 10 minutes   **Cooking time:** 15 minutes   **Servings:** 4

Ingredients:

- 1 pound chicken livers, cleaned and trimmed
- 2 tablespoons unsalted butter
- 1/4 cup heavy cream
- 1 small onion, finely chopped
- 2 cloves garlic, minced

- 1 teaspoon fresh thyme leaves
- 1/2 teaspoon salt
- 1/4 teaspoon black pepper
- 2 tablespoons brandy or cognac (optional)

Directions:

1. Preheat the air fryer to 370°F.
2. In a skillet over medium heat, melt 1 tablespoon of butter. Add the onion and garlic, sautéing until translucent, about 3-4 minutes.
3. Add the chicken livers to the skillet, cooking until they are browned on the outside but still slightly pink in the middle, approximately 5 minutes.
4. Stir in the thyme, salt, pepper, and brandy (if using), cooking for an additional 2 minutes.
5. Transfer the liver mixture to a food processor, adding the remaining butter and heavy cream. Blend until the mixture is smooth.
6. Spoon the pâté into a serving dish or individual ramekins. For best flavor, cover and refrigerate for at least 2 hours before serving.
7. Serve chilled. The pâté can be stored in the refrigerator for up to 5 days.

Per serving: Calories: 292kcal; Carbs: 4g; Fiber: 0g; Sugars: 1g; Protein: 19g; Saturated fat: 10g; Unsaturated fat: 5g.

33. Pheasant

Preparation time: 10 minutes   **Cooking time:** 20 minutes   **Servings:** 2

Ingredients:

- 1 whole pheasant, cleaned and patted dry
- 1 teaspoon salt
- 1/2 teaspoon black pepper
- 1 tablespoon olive oil
- 1/2 teaspoon thyme

Directions:

1. Preheat your air fryer to 390°F (200°C).
2. Rub the pheasant all over with olive oil. Season evenly with salt, pepper, and thyme.
3. Place the seasoned pheasant in the air fryer basket. Ensure it's positioned for even cooking.
4. Cook for 20 minutes, flipping the pheasant halfway through the cooking time to ensure it cooks evenly on all sides.
5. Check the internal temperature of the pheasant with a meat thermometer. The USDA recommends a minimum internal temperature of 165°F (74°C) for poultry.
6. Once cooked, remove the pheasant from the air fryer and let it rest for 5 minutes before carving. Resting allows the juices to redistribute, making the meat more tender and flavorful.
7. Carve the pheasant and serve immediately.

Per serving: Calories: 322kcal; Carbs: 0g; Fiber: 0g; Sugars: 0g; Protein: 48g; Saturated fat: 5g; Unsaturated fat: 7g.

34. Roasted Chicken

Preparation time: 10 minutes   **Cooking time:** 25 minutes   **Servings:** 4

Ingredients:

- 1 whole chicken (about 4 pounds)
- 2 teaspoons salt
- 1 teaspoon black pepper
- 1 teaspoon garlic powder
- 1 teaspoon onion powder
- 1 tablespoon olive oil

Directions:

1. Preheat your air fryer to 360°F (182°C).
2. Pat the chicken dry with paper towels to ensure the skin crisps up nicely.
3. Rub the chicken all over with olive oil. In a small bowl, mix together the salt, pepper, garlic powder, and onion powder. Season the chicken evenly with the spice mixture.
4. Place the chicken breast-side down in the air fryer basket. Depending on the size of your air fryer, you may need to remove the air fryer basket to fit the chicken properly.

5. Cook for 15 minutes, then carefully flip the chicken to breast-side up and cook for an additional 15 minutes, or until the internal temperature reaches 165°F (74°C) when checked with a meat thermometer inserted into the thickest part of the thigh, not touching bone.

6. Once cooked, remove the chicken from the air fryer and let it rest for 10 minutes before carving. This allows the juices to redistribute, ensuring the meat is moist and flavorful.

7. Carve the chicken and serve immediately.

Per serving: Calories: 422kcal; Carbs: 0g; Fiber: 0g; Sugars: 0g; Protein: 35g; Saturated fat: 9g; Unsaturated fat: 13g.

35. Chicken Breast with Prosciutto

Preparation time: 5 minutes   **Cooking time:** 12 minutes   **Servings:** 2

Ingredients:

- 2 small chicken breast fillets
- 4 fresh sage leaves
- 4 slices prosciutto
- Extra virgin olive oil, to drizzle
- Lemon wedges

Directions:

1. Top each 2 small chicken breast fillets piece with 4 fresh sage leaves.
2. Wrap the chicken breast with the 4 slices prosciutto to secure the leaves.
3. Place parcels, seam-side down in the air fryer.
4. Spray with Extra virgin olive oil, to drizzle.
5. Cook at 180°C for 8 minutes.
6. Place chicken on serving plates, drizzle with oil and serve with Lemon wedges.

Per serving: Calories: 270kcal; Carbs: 7g; Fiber: 1g; Sugar: 0g; Protein: 33g; Saturated fat: 2g; Unsaturated fat: 10g.

36. Chicken Heart Skewers

Preparation time: 10 minutes   **Cooking time:** 15 minutes   **Servings:** 4

Ingredients:

- 1 pound chicken hearts, cleaned and trimmed
- 1 teaspoon sea salt
- 1/2 teaspoon black pepper
- 1/2 teaspoon smoked paprika (optional for a hint of smokiness)

Directions:

1. Preheat your air fryer to 400°F (200°C).

2. In a bowl, season the chicken hearts with sea salt, black pepper, and smoked paprika (if using), ensuring they are evenly coated.

3. Thread the chicken hearts onto skewers, leaving a small space between each heart for even cooking.

4. Place the skewers in the air fryer basket, ensuring they do not touch each other.

5. Cook for 15 minutes, turning the skewers halfway through the cooking time, until the chicken hearts are fully cooked and have a slight crisp on the outside.

6. Carefully remove the skewers from the air fryer and let them rest for a few minutes before serving.

Per serving: Calories: 180kcal; Carbs: 0g; Fiber: 0g; Sugars: 0g; Protein: 26g; Saturated fat: 4g; Unsaturated fat: 3g.

Beef Recipes

37. Ribeye Steak

Preparation time: 5 minutes   **Cooking time:** 12 minutes   **Servings:** 2

Ingredients:

- 2 ribeye steaks (about 1-inch thick)
- 1 teaspoon salt
- 1/2 teaspoon black pepper
- 1/2 teaspoon garlic powder

Directions:

1. Preheat your air fryer to 400°F (200°C).
2. Season both sides of the ribeye steaks generously with salt, pepper, and garlic powder (if using).
3. Place the steaks in the air fryer basket, ensuring they are not touching to allow for even cooking.
4. Cook for 6 minutes, then flip the steaks over and cook for an additional 6 minutes for medium-rare or adjust the time according to your preferred level of doneness.
5. Once cooked to your liking, remove the steaks from the air fryer and let them rest for 3 minutes. This resting period allows the juices to redistribute throughout the meat, ensuring your steak is juicy and flavorful.
6. Serve immediately and enjoy the rich, robust flavors of your air-fried ribeye steak.

Per serving: Calories: 670kcal; Carbs: 0g; Fiber: 0g; Sugars: 0g; Protein: 50g; Saturated fat: 28g; Unsaturated fat: 30g.

38. Ground Beef Patties

Preparation time: 10 minutes   **Cooking time:** 15 minutes   **Servings:** 4

Ingredients:

- 1 pound ground beef (85% lean)
- 1 teaspoon salt
- 1/2 teaspoon black pepper

Directions:

1. Preheat your air fryer to 370°F.
2. In a bowl, mix the ground beef with salt and pepper until well combined.
3. Divide the mixture into four equal parts and shape each into a patty, about 3/4 inch thick.
4. Place the patties in the air fryer basket, ensuring they are not touching to allow for even cooking.

5. Cook for 15 minutes, flipping the patties halfway through the cooking time, until they are browned on the outside and reach your desired level of doneness.

6. Remove the patties from the air fryer and let them rest for a couple of minutes before serving.

Per serving: Calories: 278kcal; Carbs: 0g; Fiber: 0g; Sugars: 0g; Protein: 20g; Saturated fat: 10g; Unsaturated fat: 8g.

39. Beef Ribs

Preparation time: 5 minutes   **Cooking time:** 30 minutes   **Servings:** 4

Ingredients:

- 2 pounds beef ribs
- 1 tablespoon sea salt
- 1 teaspoon black pepper
- 1 teaspoon garlic powder

Directions:

1. Preheat your air fryer to 380°F (193°C).

2. Pat the beef ribs dry with paper towels to ensure proper seasoning adhesion and to help achieve a crispy texture.

3. Season the ribs evenly with sea salt, black pepper, and garlic powder. Ensure the entire surface is covered for maximum flavor.

4. Place the seasoned beef ribs in the air fryer basket. Depending on the size of your air fryer, you may need to cook them in batches to avoid overcrowding.

5. Cook for 30 minutes, flipping the ribs halfway through the cooking time to ensure they are evenly cooked and crisped on all sides.

6. Once the ribs are cooked through and have reached an internal temperature of 145°F (63°C), remove them from the air fryer and let them rest for a few minutes. This resting period allows the juices to redistribute, making the ribs even more tender and flavorful.

7. Serve hot and enjoy the succulent taste of air-fried beef ribs.

Per serving: Calories: 590kcal; Carbs: 0g; Fiber: 0g; Sugars: 0g; Protein: 58g; Saturated fat: 22g; Unsaturated fat: 25g.

40. Meatballs

Preparation time: 10 minutes   **Cooking time:** 15 minutes   **Servings:** 4

Ingredients:

- 1 pound ground beef
- 1 teaspoon salt
- 1/2 teaspoon black pepper
- 1/2 teaspoon garlic powder

Directions:

1. Preheat your air fryer to 400°F (200°C).
2. In a large bowl, combine the ground beef, salt, black pepper, and garlic powder. Mix until well combined.
3. Form the mixture into small balls, about 1 inch in diameter. This should yield approximately 16 meatballs.
4. Place the meatballs in the air fryer basket, ensuring they are not touching to allow for even cooking. You may need to cook them in batches depending on the size of your air fryer.
5. Cook for 15 minutes, or until the meatballs are browned on the outside and reach an internal temperature of 160°F (71°C).
6. Remove the meatballs from the air fryer and let them rest for a few minutes before serving.

Per serving: Calories: 276kcal; Carbs: 0g; Fiber: 0g; Sugars: 0g; Protein: 20g; Saturated fat: 9g; Unsaturated fat: 8g.

41. Beef Liver

Preparation time: 10 minutes   **Cooking time:** 8 minutes   **Servings:** 4

Ingredients:

- 1 pound beef liver, sliced into thin strips
- 1 teaspoon salt
- 1/2 teaspoon black pepper
- 1 teaspoon garlic powder

Directions:

1. Preheat your air fryer to 400°F (200°C).
2. Pat the beef liver strips dry with paper towels to remove any excess moisture. This step is crucial for achieving a crispy texture.
3. Season the liver strips evenly with salt, pepper, and garlic powder (if using).
4. Arrange the liver strips in the air fryer basket in a single layer, ensuring they are not touching to allow for even cooking.
5. Cook for 4 minutes, then flip the liver strips over and cook for an additional 4 minutes, or until they are crispy on the outside and tender on the inside.
6. Remove the beef liver from the air fryer and let it rest for a couple of minutes before serving.

Per serving: Calories: 150kcal; Carbs: 5g; Fiber: 0g; Sugars: 0g; Protein: 24g; Saturated fat: 2g; Unsaturated fat: 1g.

42. T-Bone Steak

Preparation time: 5 minutes   **Cooking time:** 15 minutes   **Servings:** 2

Ingredients:

- 2 T-Bone steaks, approximately 1 inch thick
- 1 teaspoon salt
- 1/2 teaspoon black pepper
- 1/2 teaspoon garlic powder

Directions:

1. Preheat your air fryer to 400°F (200°C).
2. Season both sides of the T-Bone steaks with salt, pepper, and garlic powder, ensuring an even coat.
3. Place the steaks in the air fryer basket, making sure they do not overlap.
4. Cook for 10 minutes, then flip the steaks and cook for an additional 5 minutes for medium-rare. Adjust the time if you prefer your steak more or less done.
5. Once cooked to your liking, remove the steaks from the air fryer and let them rest for 3 minutes. This resting period allows the juices to redistribute throughout the meat, ensuring a moist and flavorful steak.
6. Serve immediately and enjoy the rich, robust flavors of your air-fried T-Bone Steak.

Per serving: Calories: 474kcal; Carbs: 0g; Fiber: 0g; Sugars: 0g; Protein: 62g; Saturated fat: 12g; Unsaturated fat: 15g.

43. Sesame Beef Skewers

Preparation time: 15 minutes   **Cooking time:** 10 minutes   **Servings:** 4

Ingredients:

- 1 pound beef sirloin, cut into cubes
- 1 tablespoon sesame oil
- 2 cloves garlic, minced
- 1 tablespoon sesame seeds
- Salt and pepper to taste
- Wooden skewers, that is soaked in water for 30 minutes

Directions:

1. In your bowl, whisk together sesame oil, minced garlic, sesame seeds, salt, and pepper.
2. Add beef cubes to the bowl then toss to coat.
3. Thread beef cubes onto soaked wooden skewers.
4. Preheat the air fryer to 400°F.
5. Place beef skewers in your air fryer basket.

6. Air fry 8-10 minutes, turning halfway through, until beef is cooked to desired doneness.
7. Serve hot.

Per serving: Calories: 263kcal; Carbs: 5g; Fiber: 1g; Sugar: 0g; Protein: 26g; Saturated fat: 5g; Unsaturated fat: 10g.

44. Sirloin Tips

Preparation time: 5 minutes   **Cooking time:** 15 minutes   **Servings:** 4

Ingredients:

- 1 pound sirloin tips, cut into 1-inch pieces
- 1 teaspoon salt
- 1/2 teaspoon black pepper
- 1 tablespoon olive oil

Directions:

1. Preheat your air fryer to 400°F (200°C).
2. In a large bowl, toss the sirloin tips with olive oil, salt, and pepper until evenly coated.
3. Place the sirloin tips in the air fryer basket in a single layer, ensuring they are not overcrowded to allow for even cooking.
4. Cook for 15 minutes, shaking the basket halfway through the cooking time to ensure all sides of the sirloin tips are browned and cooked to perfection.
5. Once cooked, carefully remove the sirloin tips from the air fryer and let them rest for a few minutes before serving. This resting period allows the juices to redistribute, ensuring each bite is moist and flavorful.

Per serving: Calories: 210kcal; Carbs: 0g; Fiber: 0g; Sugars: 0g; Protein: 25g; Saturated fat: 3g; Unsaturated fat: 5g.

45. Parsley Garlic Steak Bites

Preparation time: 10 minutes   **Cooking time:** 10 minutes   **Servings:** 4

Ingredients:

- 1 pound beef steak (e.g., sirloin or ribeye), that is cut into bite-sized pieces
- 4 tablespoons unsalted butter, melted
- 3 cloves garlic, minced
- 1 tablespoon chopped fresh parsley
- Salt and pepper to taste

Directions:

1. In your bowl, combine melted butter, minced garlic, chopped fresh parsley, salt, and pepper.
2. Add steak pieces to the bowl then toss to coat.
3. Preheat the air fryer to 400°F.

4. Place steak pieces in your air fryer basket in a one layer.
5. Air fry 8-10 minutes, shaking the basket halfway through, until steak is cooked to desired doneness.
6. Serve hot.

Per serving: Calories: 287kcal; Carbs: 1g; Fiber: 0g; Sugar: 0g; Protein: 25g; Saturated fat: 10g; Unsaturated fat: 10g.

46. Italian Herb Crusted Beef Tenderloin

Preparation time: 10 minutes   **Cooking time:** 10 minutes   **Servings:** 4

Ingredients:

- 1 pound beef tenderloin
- 1 tablespoons olive oil
- 2 tablespoons chopped fresh herbs (e.g., rosemary, thyme, and sage)
- 2 cloves garlic, minced
- Salt and pepper to taste

Directions:

1. Preheat the air fryer to 400°F.
2. In your small bowl, mix together olive oil, chopped fresh herbs, minced garlic, salt, and pepper.
3. Rub the herb mixture over the pork tenderloin, coating it evenly.
4. Place pork tenderloin in your air fryer basket.
5. Air fry 10 minutes, flipping halfway through, until the pork is cooked through then reaches an internal temperature of 145°F.
6. Let your pork rest for a few minutes before slicing.
7. Serve hot.

Per serving: Calories: 219kcal; Carbs: 1g; Fiber: 0g; Sugar: 0g; Protein: 26g; Saturated fat: 2g; Unsaturated fat: 9g.

47. Filet Mignon

Preparation time: 5 minutes   **Cooking time:** 15 minutes   **Servings:** 2

Ingredients:

- 2 Filet Mignon steaks (about 6 ounces each)
- 1 teaspoon salt
- 1/2 teaspoon black pepper
- 1 tablespoon olive oil

Directions:

1. Preheat your air fryer to 400°F (200°C).
2. Pat the Filet Mignon steaks dry with paper towels to ensure proper seasoning and to achieve a crispy exterior.
3. Rub each steak with olive oil, then season evenly with salt and pepper.
4. Place the seasoned steaks in the air fryer basket, making sure they are not touching to allow for even cooking.
5. Cook for 6 minutes, then flip the steaks over and cook for an additional 6 minutes for medium-rare, or adjust the time according to your preferred level of doneness.
6. Once cooked, remove the steaks from the air fryer and let them rest for 3-5 minutes before serving. Resting allows the juices to redistribute throughout the meat, ensuring each bite is as flavorful as possible.
7. Serve the Filet Mignon steaks as is or with your favorite carnivore diet-approved sides.

Per serving: Calories: 390kcal; Carbs: 0g; Fiber: 0g; Sugars: 0g; Protein: 23g; Saturated fat: 14g; Unsaturated fat: 18g.

48. Mediterranean Beef Skewers

Preparation time: 10 minutes   **Cooking time:** 20 minutes   **Servings:** 4

Ingredients:

- 1 pound lean beef, cut into cubes
- 1 teaspoon onion powder
- 1 tablespoons olive oil
- 1 teaspoon dried oregano
- 1 teaspoon ground cumin
- Salt and pepper to taste

Directions:

1. In your bowl, combine beef, onion powder, olive oil, dried oregano, ground cumin, salt, and pepper.
2. Thread the beef onto skewers.
3. Preheat your air fryer to 375°F.
4. Place the kebabs in your air fryer basket.
5. Cook for 18-20 minutes, turning occasionally, 'til the beef is cooked to your wanted level of doneness.
6. Serve hot.

Per serving: Calories: 180kcal; Carbs: 0g; Fiber: 0g; Sugars: 0g; Protein: 20g; Saturated fat: 6g; Unsaturated fat: 4g.

Lamb Recipes

49. Lamb Shoulder

Preparation time: 5 minutes   **Cooking time:** 35 minutes   **Servings:** 4

Ingredients:

- 1 lamb shoulder (about 3-4 pounds)
- 2 teaspoons salt
- 1 teaspoon black pepper
- 1 teaspoon rosemary

Directions:

1. Preheat your air fryer to 360°F (182°C).
2. Pat the lamb shoulder dry with paper towels to ensure proper seasoning adhesion.
3. Season the lamb shoulder evenly with salt, pepper, and rosemary, ensuring full coverage.
4. Place the seasoned lamb shoulder in the air fryer basket.
5. Cook for 35 minutes, or until the lamb is tender and easily pulls apart with a fork. For larger cuts, adjust cooking time accordingly.
6. Once cooked, remove the lamb shoulder from the air fryer and let it rest for 10 minutes before serving. This resting period allows the juices to redistribute, ensuring the meat is moist and flavorful.
7. Carve the lamb shoulder and serve immediately.

Per serving: Calories: 310kcal; Carbs: 0g; Fiber: 0g; Sugars: 0g; Protein: 47g; Saturated fat: 8g; Unsaturated fat: 11g.

50. Rack of Lamb

Preparation time: 10 minutes   **Cooking time:** 22 minutes   **Servings:** 2

Ingredients:

- 1 rack of lamb (about 1.5 pounds), trimmed
- 1 teaspoon salt
- 1/2 teaspoon black pepper
- 1 tablespoon olive oil
- 1/2 teaspoon rosemary, finely chopped

Directions:

1. Preheat your air fryer to 400°F (200°C).
2. Pat the rack of lamb dry with paper towels. This will help to achieve a better sear.

3. Rub the entire rack with olive oil, then season evenly with salt, pepper, and rosemary.

4. Place the rack of lamb in the air fryer basket, meaty side up.

5. Cook for 22 minutes, or until the internal temperature reaches 135°F (57°C) for medium-rare. Adjust the cooking time if you prefer your lamb more or less done.

6. Once cooked, remove the rack of lamb from the air fryer and let it rest for 5 minutes before carving. Resting allows the juices to redistribute throughout the meat, ensuring each bite is moist and flavorful.

7. Slice between the ribs and serve immediately.

Per serving: Calories: 410kcal; Carbs: 0g; Fiber: 0g; Sugars: 0g; Protein: 40g; Saturated fat: 14g; Unsaturated fat: 18g.

51. Lamb Burgers

Preparation time: 10 minutes   **Cooking time:** 15 minutes   **Servings:** 4

Ingredients:

- 1 pound ground lamb
- 1 teaspoon salt
- 1/2 teaspoon black pepper
- 1/2 teaspoon rosemary, finely chopped

Directions:

1. Preheat your air fryer to 370°F (187°C).

2. In a large bowl, combine the ground lamb, salt, pepper, and rosemary (if using). Mix the ingredients until well combined.

3. Divide the mixture into four equal portions. Shape each portion into a burger patty, about 3/4 inch thick.

4. Place the lamb patties in the air fryer basket, ensuring they are not touching to allow for even cooking.

5. Cook for 15 minutes, flipping the patties halfway through the cooking time, or until they reach your desired level of doneness.

6. Once cooked, remove the lamb burgers from the air fryer and let them rest for a couple of minutes before serving.

Per serving: Calories: 330kcal; Carbs: 0g; Fiber: 0g; Sugars: 0g; Protein: 20g; Saturated fat: 16g; Unsaturated fat: 13g

52. Lamb Ribs

Preparation time: 10 minutes   **Cooking time:** 20 minutes   **Servings:** 4

Ingredients:

- 2 pounds lamb ribs
- 1 teaspoon salt
- 1/2 teaspoon black pepper
- 1/2 teaspoon rosemary

Directions:

1. Preheat your air fryer to 380°F (193°C).
2. Pat the lamb ribs dry with paper towels to ensure proper seasoning adhesion and to help achieve a crispy texture.
3. Season the ribs evenly with salt, pepper, and rosemary. Ensure the entire surface is covered for maximum flavor.
4. Place the seasoned lamb ribs in the air fryer basket. Depending on the size of your air fryer, you may need to cook them in batches to avoid overcrowding.
5. Cook for 20 minutes, flipping the ribs halfway through the cooking time to ensure they are evenly cooked and crisped on all sides.
6. Once the ribs are cooked through and have reached an internal temperature of 145°F (63°C), remove them from the air fryer and let them rest for a few minutes. This resting period allows the juices to redistribute, making the ribs even more tender and flavorful.
7. Serve hot and enjoy the succulent taste of air-fried lamb ribs.

Per serving: Calories: 310kcal; Carbs: 0g; Fiber: 0g; Sugars: 0g; Protein: 25g; Saturated fat: 14g; Unsaturated fat: 12g.

53. Ground Lamb

Preparation time: 10 minutes   **Cooking time:** 10 minutes   **Servings:** 4

Ingredients:

- 1 pound ground lamb
- 1 teaspoon sea salt
- 1/2 teaspoon black pepper

Directions:

1. Preheat your air fryer to 400°F (200°C).
2. In a large bowl, mix the ground lamb with sea salt and black pepper until well combined.
3. Divide the mixture into four equal parts and shape each into a patty, about 3/4 inch thick.
4. Place the patties in the air fryer basket, ensuring they are not touching to allow for even cooking.

5. Cook for 10 minutes, flipping the patties halfway through the cooking time, until they are browned on the outside and reach your desired level of doneness.

6. Remove the patties from the air fryer and let them rest for a couple of minutes before serving.

Per serving: Calories: 330kcal; Carbs: 0g; Fiber: 0g; Sugars: 0g; Protein: 19g; Saturated fat: 15g; Unsaturated fat: 13g.

54. Lamb Heart

Preparation time: 10 minutes   **Cooking time:** 15 minutes   **Servings:** 2

Ingredients:

- 2 lamb hearts, trimmed and sliced into 1/4-inch thick pieces
- 1 teaspoon salt
- 1/2 teaspoon black pepper

Directions:

1. Preheat your air fryer to 380°F (193°C).

2. Pat the lamb heart slices dry with paper towels to remove any excess moisture. This step is crucial for achieving a crispy texture.

3. Season the lamb heart slices evenly with salt and pepper.

4. Arrange the slices in a single layer in the air fryer basket, ensuring they are not touching to allow for even cooking.

5. Cook for 15 minutes, flipping the slices halfway through the cooking time, until they are cooked through and slightly crispy on the edges.

6. Remove the lamb heart slices from the air fryer and let them rest for a couple of minutes before serving. This resting period allows the juices to redistribute, ensuring each bite is moist and flavorful.

Per serving: Calories: 250kcal; Carbs: 0g; Fiber: 0g; Sugars: 0g; Protein: 38g; Saturated fat: 4g; Unsaturated fat: 2g.

55. Lamb Sausages

Preparation time: 15 minutes   **Cooking time:** 10 minutes   **Servings:** 4

Ingredients:

- 1 pound ground lamb
- 1 teaspoon sea salt
- 1/2 teaspoon black pepper
- 1 teaspoon dried rosemary
- 1/2 teaspoon dried thyme
- 1/4 teaspoon garlic powder

Directions:

1. In a large mixing bowl, combine the ground lamb, sea salt, black pepper, dried rosemary, dried thyme, and garlic powder. Mix thoroughly until all the spices are evenly distributed throughout the lamb.
2. Divide the mixture into equal portions and shape each portion into a sausage link, about 4 inches long and 1 inch thick.
3. Preheat your air fryer to 400°F (200°C).
4. Place the lamb sausages in the air fryer basket, ensuring they are not touching to allow for even cooking.
5. Cook for 10 minutes, turning the sausages halfway through the cooking time, until they are browned on the outside and cooked through.
6. Carefully remove the lamb sausages from the air fryer and let them rest for a couple of minutes before serving.

Per serving: Calories: 282kcal; Carbs: 0g; Fiber: 0g; Sugars: 0g; Protein: 19g; Saturated fat: 12g; Unsaturated fat: 9g.

56. Lamb Steaks

Preparation time: 5 minutes   **Cooking time:** 12 minutes   **Servings:** 2

Ingredients:

- 2 lamb steaks (about 1-inch thick)
- 1 teaspoon salt
- 1/2 teaspoon black pepper
- 1 tablespoon olive oil

Directions:

1. Preheat your air fryer to 400°F (200°C).
2. Rub each lamb steak with olive oil, then season both sides generously with salt and pepper.
3. Place the lamb steaks in the air fryer basket, ensuring they are not touching to allow for even cooking.
4. Cook for 6 minutes, then flip the steaks over and cook for an additional 6 minutes for medium-rare, or adjust the time according to your preferred level of doneness.
5. Once cooked to your liking, remove the lamb steaks from the air fryer and let them rest for 3 minutes. This resting period allows the juices to redistribute throughout the meat, ensuring your steak is juicy and flavorful.
6. Serve the lamb steaks immediately, enjoying the rich and tender flavors that make lamb a carnivore diet favorite.

Per serving: Calories: 320kcal; Carbs: 0g; Fiber: 0g; Sugars: 0g; Protein: 24g; Saturated fat: 10g; Unsaturated fat: 13g.

57. Lamb Kidney

Preparation time: 10 minutes   **Cooking time:** 8 minutes   **Servings:** 2

Ingredients:

- 4 lamb kidneys, cleaned and halved
- 1 teaspoon salt
- 1/2 teaspoon black pepper
- 1 tablespoon olive oil

Directions:

1. Preheat your air fryer to 400°F (200°C).
2. Pat the lamb kidneys dry with paper towels to ensure they cook evenly.
3. Season the kidneys with salt and pepper, then lightly coat them with olive oil.
4. Arrange the kidneys in the air fryer basket, ensuring they are not touching to allow for even cooking.
5. Cook for 4 minutes, then flip the kidneys over and cook for an additional 4 minutes, or until they are browned on the outside and tender on the inside.
6. Remove the kidneys from the air fryer and let them rest for a couple of minutes before serving.

Per serving: Calories: 210kcal; Carbs: 0g; Fiber: 0g; Sugars: 0g; Protein: 27g; Saturated fat: 3g; Unsaturated fat: 5g.

58. Lamb Liver

Preparation time: 10 minutes   **Cooking time:** 8 minutes   **Servings:** 2

Ingredients:

- 1 pound lamb liver, sliced into thin strips
- 1 teaspoon sea salt
- 1/2 teaspoon black pepper
- 1/2 teaspoon dried rosemary

Directions:

1. Preheat your air fryer to 380°F (193°C).
2. Pat the lamb liver strips dry with paper towels to remove any excess moisture. This step is crucial for achieving a crispy texture.
3. Season the liver strips evenly with sea salt, black pepper, and dried rosemary (if using).
4. Arrange the liver strips in the air fryer basket in a single layer, ensuring they are not touching to allow for even cooking.
5. Cook for 4 minutes, then gently flip the liver strips over and cook for an additional 4 minutes, or until they are crispy on the outside and tender on the inside.
6. Carefully remove the lamb liver from the air fryer and let it rest for a couple of minutes before serving.

Per serving: Calories: 192kcal; Carbs: 5g; Fiber: 0g; Sugars: 0g; Protein: 27g; Saturated fat: 2g; Unsaturated fat: 1g.

59. Lamb Meatballs

Preparation time: 10 minutes   **Cooking time:** 15 minutes   **Servings:** 4

Ingredients:

- 1 pound ground lamb
- 1 teaspoon salt
- 1/2 teaspoon black pepper
- 1/2 teaspoon rosemary, finely chopped

Directions:

1. Preheat your air fryer to 400°F (200°C).

2. In a large bowl, combine the ground lamb, salt, black pepper, and rosemary (if using). Mix well until all the ingredients are evenly distributed.

3. Form the mixture into small balls, about 1 inch in diameter, to make the meatballs.

4. Place the meatballs in the air fryer basket, ensuring they are not touching to allow for even cooking. You may need to cook in batches depending on the size of your air fryer.

5. Cook for 15 minutes, or until the meatballs are browned on the outside and cooked through.

6. Remove the meatballs from the air fryer and let them rest for a couple of minutes before serving.

Per serving: Calories: 330kcal; Carbs: 0g; Fiber: 0g; Sugars: 0g; Protein: 20g; Saturated fat: 15g; Unsaturated fat: 13g.

60. Spiced Lamb Chops

Preparation time: 5 minutes   **Cooking time:** 15 minutes   **Servings:** 2

Ingredients:

- 4 lamb chops, about 1 inch thick
- 1 teaspoon salt
- 1/2 teaspoon black pepper
- 1/2 teaspoon cumin
- 1/2 teaspoon smoked paprika
- 1/4 teaspoon garlic powder
- 1 tablespoon olive oil

Directions:

1. Preheat your air fryer to 400°F (200°C).

2. In a small bowl, mix together salt, black pepper, cumin, smoked paprika, and garlic powder.

3. Rub each lamb chop with olive oil, then evenly coat with the spice mixture.

4. Place the lamb chops in the air fryer basket, ensuring they are not touching to allow for even cooking.

5. Cook for 15 minutes, flipping the chops halfway through the cooking time, until they are well-browned on the outside and reach your desired level of doneness.

6. Remove the lamb chops from the air fryer and let them rest for 3 minutes before serving. This resting period allows the juices to redistribute, ensuring each chop is moist and flavorful.

Per serving: Calories: 310kcal; Carbs: 1g; Fiber: 0g; Sugars: 0g; Protein: 25g; Saturated fat: 7g; Unsaturated fat: 5g.

Seafood and Fish Recipes

61. Salmon Steaks

Preparation time: 5 minutes   **Cooking time:** 10 minutes   **Servings:** 2

Ingredients:

- 2 salmon steaks (about 6 ounces each)
- 1 teaspoon salt
- 1/2 teaspoon black pepper
- 1 tablespoon olive oil

Directions:

1. Preheat your air fryer to 400°F (200°C).
2. Season the salmon steaks on both sides with salt and pepper.
3. Rub each steak with olive oil to ensure an even cook and a crispy exterior.
4. Place the salmon steaks in the air fryer basket, making sure they are not touching to allow for even air circulation.
5. Cook for 10 minutes, or until the salmon is cooked through and flakes easily with a fork. There's no need to flip the steaks halfway through.
6. Once cooked, carefully remove the salmon steaks from the air fryer and let them rest for a couple of minutes before serving. This resting period allows the juices to redistribute, ensuring each bite is moist and flavorful.

Per serving: Calories: 280kcal; Carbs: 0g; Fiber: 0g; Sugars: 0g; Protein: 34g; Saturated fat: 4g; Unsaturated fat: 10g.

62. Tuna Steaks

Preparation time: 5 minutes   **Cooking time:** 10 minutes   **Servings:** 2

Ingredients:

- 2 tuna steaks (6 ounces each)
- 1 tablespoon olive oil
- Salt and pepper to taste
- Optional: Lemon wedges and fresh dill for garnish

Directions:

1. Preheat your air fryer to 400°F (200°C).
2. Pat the tuna steaks dry with paper towels. This step is crucial for getting that perfect sear.

3. Rub each fillet with olive oil, then season generously with salt and pepper. If you're feeling adventurous, a sprinkle of your favorite herbs can add an extra layer of flavor.

4. Place the tuna steaks in the air fryer basket, ensuring they are not touching to allow for even cooking.

5. Cook for 10 minutes, or until the tuna easily flakes with a fork. There's no need to flip the fillets halfway through.

6. Once done, carefully remove the tuna from the air fryer and let it rest for a couple of minutes. This rest period lets the juices redistribute, ensuring your tuna is moist and flavorful.

7. Serve immediately, garnished with lemon wedges and fresh dill if desired.

Per serving: Calories: 280kcal; Carbs: 0g; Fiber: 0g; Sugars: 0g; Protein: 34g; Saturated fat: 4g; Unsaturated fat: 10g.

63. Air-Fried Shrimp

Preparation time: 5 minutes   **Cooking time:** 8 minutes   **Servings:** 4

Ingredients:

- 1 pound large shrimp, peeled and deveined
- 1 teaspoon salt
- 1/2 teaspoon black pepper
- 1/2 teaspoon garlic powder
- 1 tablespoon olive oil

Directions:

1. Preheat your air fryer to 400°F (200°C).

2. In a large bowl, toss the shrimp with olive oil, salt, black pepper, and garlic powder until they are evenly coated.

3. Arrange the shrimp in a single layer in the air fryer basket, ensuring they are not touching to allow for even cooking.

4. Cook for 8 minutes, flipping the shrimp halfway through the cooking time, until they are golden brown and cooked through.

5. Once cooked, carefully remove the shrimp from the air fryer and let them rest for a minute before serving.

Per serving: Calories: 120kcal; Carbs: 1g; Fiber: 0g; Sugars: 0g; Protein: 23g; Saturated fat: 1g; Unsaturated fat: 2g.

64. Lobster Tails

Preparation time: 10 minutes   **Cooking time:** 8 minutes   **Servings:** 2

Ingredients:

- 2 lobster tails
- 1 tablespoon olive oil
- Salt and pepper to taste

Directions:

1. Preheat your air fryer to 380°F (193°C).
2. Using kitchen shears, cut down the center of the lobster tail shells lengthwise. Gently pry open the shell to expose the meat.
3. Brush the lobster meat with olive oil and season with salt and black pepper.
4. Place the lobster tails in the air fryer basket, meat side up, ensuring they are not touching.
5. Cook for 8 minutes, or until the lobster meat is opaque and cooked through.
6. Remove the lobster tails from the air fryer and let them rest for a couple of minutes before serving.

Per serving: Calories: 143kcal; Carbs: 0g; Fiber: 0g; Sugars: 0g; Protein: 20g; Saturated fat: 1g; Unsaturated fat: 5g.

65. Cod Fillets

Preparation time: 5 minutes   **Cooking time:** 12 minutes   **Servings:** 2

Ingredients:

- 2 cod fillets (6 ounces each)
- 1 teaspoon salt
- 1/2 teaspoon black pepper
- 1 tablespoon olive oil

Directions:

1. Preheat your air fryer to 400°F (200°C).
2. Pat the cod fillets dry with paper towels to remove any excess moisture. This step is crucial for achieving a perfectly cooked fillet.
3. Rub each fillet with olive oil, then season evenly with salt and pepper.
4. Place the cod fillets in the air fryer basket, ensuring they are not touching to allow for even cooking.
5. Cook for 12 minutes, or until the cod fillets are flaky and opaque throughout.
6. Remove the cod fillets from the air fryer and let them rest for a couple of minutes before serving.

Per serving: Calories: 190kcal; Carbs: 0g; Fiber: 0g; Sugars: 0g; Protein: 31g; Saturated fat: 1g; Unsaturated fat: 3g.

66. Air-Fried Sardines

Preparation time: 5 minutes   **Cooking time:** 10 minutes   **Servings:** 2

Ingredients:

- 1 pound fresh sardines, cleaned and gutted
- 1 teaspoon sea salt
- 1/2 teaspoon black pepper
- 1 tablespoon olive oil

Directions:

1. Preheat your air fryer to 400°F (200°C).
2. Pat the sardines dry with paper towels to remove any excess moisture. This step is crucial for achieving a crispy texture.
3. In a small bowl, mix together the sea salt and black pepper.
4. Lightly brush each sardine with olive oil, then evenly sprinkle the salt and pepper mixture over them.
5. Arrange the sardines in the air fryer basket in a single layer, ensuring they are not touching to allow for even cooking.
6. Cook for 10 minutes, or until the sardines are golden brown and crispy.
7. Remove the sardines from the air fryer and let them rest for a couple of minutes before serving.

Per serving: Calories: 220kcal; Carbs: 0g; Fiber: 0g; Sugars: 0g; Protein: 25g; Saturated fat: 3g; Unsaturated fat: 5g.

67. Air-Fried Mackerel

Preparation time: 5 minutes   **Cooking time:** 10 minutes   **Servings:** 2

Ingredients:

- 2 whole mackerel, cleaned and gutted
- 1 teaspoon salt
- 1/2 teaspoon black pepper
- 1 tablespoon olive oil

Directions:

1. Preheat your air fryer to 400°F (200°C).
2. Pat the mackerel dry with paper towels to ensure the skin crisps up nicely.
3. Rub each mackerel with olive oil, then season both sides generously with salt and pepper.
4. Place the mackerel in the air fryer basket, ensuring they are not touching to allow for even cooking.
5. Cook for 10 minutes, or until the skin is crispy and the flesh flakes easily with a fork.
6. Carefully remove the mackerel from the air fryer and let them rest for a couple of minutes before serving.

Per serving: Calories: 310kcal; Carbs: 0g; Fiber: 0g; Sugars: 0g; Protein: 22g; Saturated fat: 5g; Unsaturated fat: 10g.

68. Crab Legs

Preparation time: 5 minutes   **Cooking time:** 10 minutes   **Servings:** 2

Ingredients:

- 1 pound crab legs, thawed if frozen
- 1 tablespoon olive oil
- 1/2 teaspoon salt
- 1/4 teaspoon black pepper

Directions:

1. Preheat your air fryer to 375°F (190°C).
2. Brush the crab legs lightly with olive oil, then season with salt and pepper.
3. Arrange the crab legs in the air fryer basket, ensuring they are not overcrowded for even cooking. You may need to cook them in batches depending on the size of your air fryer.
4. Cook for 10 minutes, flipping halfway through, until the crab legs are heated through and slightly crispy on the outside.
5. Carefully remove the crab legs from the air fryer and serve immediately with your choice of carnivore diet-approved dipping sauces or simply enjoy the natural flavors of the crab.

Per serving: Calories: 130kcal; Carbs: 0g; Fiber: 0g; Sugars: 0g; Protein: 25g; Saturated fat: 0g; Unsaturated fat: 2g.

69. Air-Fried Scallops

Preparation time: 5 minutes   **Cooking time:** 10 minutes   **Servings:** 2

Ingredients:

- 1 pound fresh scallops
- 1 teaspoon olive oil
- 1/2 teaspoon salt
- 1/4 teaspoon black pepper

Directions:

1. Preheat your air fryer to 400°F (200°C).
2. Pat the scallops dry with paper towels to remove any excess moisture. This step is crucial for achieving a golden, crispy exterior.
3. Toss the scallops with olive oil, salt, and pepper in a bowl, ensuring they are evenly coated.
4. Arrange the scallops in a single layer in the air fryer basket, making sure they are not touching to allow for even cooking.
5. Cook for 10 minutes, flipping the scallops halfway through the cooking time, until they are golden brown on the outside and opaque in the center.
6. Carefully remove the scallops from the air fryer and let them rest for a minute before serving.

Per serving: Calories: 200kcal; Carbs: 5g; Fiber: 0g; Sugars: 0g; Protein: 37g; Saturated fat: 0.5g; Unsaturated fat: 1g.

70. Air-Fried Oysters

Preparation time: 10 minutes   **Cooking time:** 6 minutes   **Servings:** 2

Ingredients:

- 12 fresh oysters, shucked
- 1 tablespoon olive oil
- Salt and black pepper to taste

Directions:

1. Preheat your air fryer to 400°F (200°C).
2. Pat the oysters dry with paper towels to remove any excess moisture. This step is crucial for achieving a crispy texture.
3. Lightly brush each oyster with olive oil, then season with salt and black pepper.
4. Arrange the oysters in the air fryer basket in a single layer, ensuring they are not touching to allow for even cooking.
5. Cook for 6 minutes, or until the oysters are golden brown and crispy.
6. Carefully remove the oysters from the air fryer and let them rest for a minute before serving.

Per serving: Calories: 157kcal; Carbs: 7g; Fiber: 0g; Sugars: 0g; Protein: 10g; Saturated fat: 1g; Unsaturated fat: 5g.

71. Air-Fried Halibut

Preparation time: 5 minutes   **Cooking time:** 12 minutes   **Servings:** 2

Ingredients:

- 2 halibut fillets (6 ounces each)
- 1 teaspoon salt
- 1/2 teaspoon black pepper
- 1 tablespoon olive oil

Directions:

1. Preheat your air fryer to 400°F (200°C).
2. Pat the halibut fillets dry with paper towels to remove any excess moisture. This step is crucial for achieving a crispy finish.
3. Rub each fillet with olive oil, then season evenly with salt and pepper.
4. Place the seasoned halibut fillets in the air fryer basket, ensuring they are not touching to allow for even cooking.
5. Cook for 12 minutes, or until the halibut is cooked through and the exterior is slightly golden and crispy.
6. Carefully remove the halibut fillets from the air fryer and let them rest for a couple of minutes before serving.

Per serving: Calories: 220kcal; Carbs: 0g; Fiber: 0g; Sugars: 0g; Protein: 31g; Saturated fat: 2g; Unsaturated fat: 5g.

72. Air-Fried Swordfish Steaks

Preparation time: 5 minutes   **Cooking time:** 10 minutes   **Servings:** 2

Ingredients:

- 2 swordfish steaks (about 6 ounces each)
- 1 teaspoon salt
- 1/2 teaspoon black pepper
- 1 tablespoon olive oil

Directions:

1. Preheat your air fryer to 400°F (200°C).
2. Pat the swordfish steaks dry with paper towels to ensure proper seasoning adhesion and to achieve a crispy exterior.
3. Rub each steak with olive oil, then season both sides generously with salt and pepper.
4. Place the swordfish steaks in the air fryer basket, ensuring they are not touching to allow for even cooking.
5. Cook for 10 minutes, flipping the steaks halfway through the cooking time, until they are well-browned on the outside and reach an internal temperature of 145°F (63°C).
6. Once cooked, remove the swordfish steaks from the air fryer and let them rest for 3 minutes before serving. This resting period allows the juices to redistribute, ensuring each steak is moist and flavorful.
7. Serve the swordfish steaks immediately, enjoying the rich and tender flavors that make swordfish a carnivore diet favorite.

Per serving: Calories: 280kcal; Carbs: 0g; Fiber: 0g; Sugars: 0g; Protein: 34g; Saturated fat: 4g; Unsaturated fat: 10g.

Game and Offal Recipes

73. Venison Steak

Preparation time: 5 minutes   **Cooking time:** 12 minutes   **Servings:** 2

Ingredients:

- 2 venison steaks (about 6 ounces each)
- 1 teaspoon salt
- 1/2 teaspoon black pepper
- 1 tablespoon olive oil

Directions:

1. Preheat your air fryer to 400°F (200°C).
2. Pat the venison steaks dry with paper towels to ensure proper seasoning adhesion and to achieve a crispy exterior.
3. Rub each steak with olive oil, then season both sides generously with salt and pepper.
4. Place the venison steaks in the air fryer basket, ensuring they are not touching to allow for even cooking.
5. Cook for 6 minutes, then flip the steaks over and cook for an additional 6 minutes for medium-rare, or adjust the time according to your preferred level of doneness.
6. Once cooked, remove the venison steaks from the air fryer and let them rest for 3 minutes before serving. This resting period allows the juices to redistribute, ensuring each steak is moist and flavorful.
7. Serve the venison steaks immediately, savoring the rich and tender flavors that make venison a carnivore diet favorite.

Per serving: Calories: 280kcal; Carbs: 0g; Fiber: 0g; Sugars: 0g; Protein: 34g; Saturated fat: 4g; Unsaturated fat: 10g.

74. Black and White Liver

Preparation time: 5 minutes   **Cooking time:** 12 minutes   **Servings:** 4

Ingredients:

- 1 pound beef liver
- 1 teaspoon onion powder
- 3/4 teaspoon salt
- 1/4 teaspoon black pepper
- 1 tablespoon olive oil

Directions:

1. Preheat your air fryer to 400°F (200°F).
2. In the meantime, slice the liver into thin slices.
3. Rub the slices liver steak with olive oil, then season both sides generously with onion powder, salt and black pepper
4. Add liver and onion mixture to the air fryer.
5. Cook liver in the air fryer at 400°F (200°C) for 12 minutes, mixing with thoroughly halfway through the cooking time.
6. Serve hot.

Per serving: Calories: 164kcal; Carbs: 7g; Fiber 0g; Sugars: 0g; Protein: 23g; Saturated fat: 1g; Unsaturated fat: 3g.

75. Elk Burgers

Preparation time: 10 minutes   **Cooking time:** 10 minutes   **Servings:** 4

Ingredients:

- 1 pound ground elk meat
- 1 teaspoon salt
- 1/2 teaspoon black pepper
- 1/2 teaspoon garlic powder

Directions:

1. Preheat your air fryer to 375°F (190°C).
2. In a large bowl, mix the ground elk meat with salt, black pepper, and garlic powder until well combined.
3. Divide the mixture into four equal portions and shape each into a burger patty, about 3/4 inch thick.
4. Place the patties in the air fryer basket, ensuring they are not touching to allow for even cooking.
5. Cook for 10 minutes, flipping the patties halfway through the cooking time, or until they reach your desired level of doneness.
6. Once cooked, remove the elk burgers from the air fryer and let them rest for a couple of minutes before serving.

Per serving: Calories: 224kcal; Carbs: 0g; Fiber: 0g; Sugars: 0g; Protein: 32g; Saturated fat: 3g; Unsaturated fat: 1g.

76. Bison Ribs

Preparation time: 5 minutes   **Cooking time:** 35 minutes   **Servings:** 4

Ingredients:

- 2 pounds bison ribs
- 1 tablespoon sea salt
- 1 teaspoon black pepper
- 1/2 teaspoon garlic powder

Directions:

1. Preheat your air fryer to 380°F (193°C).
2. Pat the bison ribs dry with paper towels to ensure proper seasoning adhesion and to help achieve a crispy texture.
3. Season the ribs evenly with sea salt, black pepper, and garlic powder. Ensure the entire surface is covered for maximum flavor.
4. Place the seasoned bison ribs in the air fryer basket. Depending on the size of your air fryer, you may need to cook them in batches to avoid overcrowding.
5. Cook for 35 minutes, flipping the ribs halfway through the cooking time to ensure they are evenly cooked and crisped on all sides.
6. Once the ribs are cooked through and have reached an internal temperature of 145°F (63°C), remove them from the air fryer and let them rest for a few minutes. This resting period allows the juices to redistribute, making the ribs even more tender and flavorful.
7. Serve hot and enjoy the succulent taste of air-fried bison ribs.

Per serving: Calories: 590kcal; Carbs: 0g; Fiber: 0g; Sugars: 0g; Protein: 58g; Saturated fat: 22g; Unsaturated fat: 25g.

77. Duck Liver

Preparation time: 5 minutes   **Cooking time:** 8 minutes   **Servings:** 2

Ingredients:

- 1/2 pound duck liver, cleaned and trimmed
- 1 tablespoon unsalted butter, melted
- Salt and pepper to taste

Directions:

1. Preheat your air fryer to 360°F (182°C).
2. Pat the duck liver dry with paper towels to remove any excess moisture. This step is crucial for achieving a tender texture.
3. Season the duck liver generously with salt and pepper, then lightly coat with melted butter to enhance the flavor and facilitate cooking.

4. Arrange the seasoned duck liver in the air fryer basket in a single layer, ensuring they are not overlapping.

5. Cook for 8 minutes, or until the duck liver is cooked through yet still tender on the inside. There's no need to flip them halfway through.

6. Carefully remove the duck liver from the air fryer and let it rest for a couple of minutes before serving. This resting period allows the flavors to meld and intensify.

Per serving: Calories: 150kcal; Carbs: 1g; Fiber: 0g; Sugars: 0g; Protein: 22g; Saturated fat: 5g; Unsaturated fat: 3g.

78. Air-Fried Pheasant

Preparation time: 10 minutes   **Cooking time:** 20 minutes   **Servings:** 2

Ingredients:

- 1 whole pheasant, cleaned and patted dry
- 1 teaspoon salt
- 1/2 teaspoon black pepper
- 1 tablespoon olive oil

Directions:

1. Preheat your air fryer to 390°F (200°C).
2. Rub the pheasant all over with olive oil. Season evenly with salt and pepper.
3. Place the seasoned pheasant in the air fryer basket. Ensure it's positioned for even cooking.
4. Cook for 20 minutes, flipping the pheasant halfway through the cooking time to ensure it cooks evenly on all sides.
5. Check the internal temperature of the pheasant with a meat thermometer. The USDA recommends a minimum internal temperature of 165°F (74°C) for poultry.
6. Once cooked, remove the pheasant from the air fryer and let it rest for 5 minutes before carving. Resting allows the juices to redistribute, making the meat more tender and flavorful.
7. Carve the pheasant and serve immediately.

Per serving: Calories: 322kcal; Carbs: 0g; Fiber: 0g; Sugars: 0g; Protein: 48g; Saturated fat: 5g; Unsaturated fat: 7g.

79. Quail Eggs

Preparation time: 5 minutes   **Cooking time:** 5 minutes   **Servings:** 2

Ingredients:

- 12 quail eggs
- Salt and black pepper to taste

Directions:

1. Preheat your air fryer to 390°F (200°C).
2. Carefully place the quail eggs in the air fryer basket, ensuring they are not touching to allow for even cooking.
3. Cook for 5 minutes for soft-boiled eggs or adjust the time up to 8 minutes for hard-boiled eggs, depending on your preference.
4. Once cooked, use a spoon to carefully remove the quail eggs from the air fryer and place them into a bowl of ice water for a minute to stop the cooking process.
5. Peel the quail eggs, season with salt and pepper to taste, and serve immediately.

Per serving: Calories: 42kcal; Carbs: 0g; Fiber: 0g; Sugars: 0g; Protein: 4g; Saturated fat: 1g; Unsaturated fat: 1g.

80. Moose Meatballs

Preparation time: 15 minutes   **Cooking time:** 15 minutes   **Servings:** 4

Ingredients:

- 1 pound ground moose meat
- 1 teaspoon salt
- 1/2 teaspoon black pepper
- 1/2 teaspoon garlic powder
- 1/2 teaspoon onion powder
- 1 tablespoon olive oil

Directions:

1. In a large mixing bowl, combine the ground moose meat with salt, black pepper, garlic powder, and onion powder. Mix thoroughly until all the ingredients are evenly distributed throughout the meat.
2. Form the mixture into small balls, about 1 inch in diameter, to create the meatballs.
3. Preheat your air fryer to 400°F (200°C).
4. Lightly brush each meatball with olive oil to ensure a crispy finish.
5. Place the meatballs in the air fryer basket, making sure they are not touching to allow for even cooking. You may need to cook them in batches depending on the size of your air fryer.
6. Cook for 15 minutes, or until the meatballs are browned on the outside and cooked through.
7. Carefully remove the meatballs from the air fryer and let them rest for a couple of minutes before serving.

Per serving: Calories: 280kcal; Carbs: 0g; Fiber: 0g; Sugars: 0g; Protein: 22g; Saturated fat: 5g; Unsaturated fat: 3g.

81. Bear Steak

Preparation time: 10 minutes   **Cooking time:** 15 minutes   **Servings:** 2

Ingredients:

- 2 bear steaks (about 6 ounces each)
- 1 teaspoon salt
- 1/2 teaspoon black pepper
- 1 tablespoon olive oil

Directions:

1. Preheat your air fryer to 400°F (200°C).
2. Pat the bear steaks dry with paper towels to ensure proper seasoning adhesion and to achieve a crispy exterior.
3. Rub each steak with olive oil, then season both sides generously with salt and pepper.
4. Place the bear steaks in the air fryer basket, ensuring they are not touching to allow for even cooking.
5. Cook for 15 minutes, flipping the steaks halfway through the cooking time, until they are well-browned on the outside and reach an internal temperature of 145°F (63°C) for medium-rare.
6. Once cooked, remove the bear steaks from the air fryer and let them rest for 3 minutes before serving. This resting period allows the juices to redistribute, ensuring each steak is moist and flavorful.
7. Serve the bear steaks immediately, enjoying the unique and rich flavors that make bear meat a carnivore diet delicacy.

Per serving: Calories: 320kcal; Carbs: 0g; Fiber: 0g; Sugars: 0g; Protein: 34g; Saturated fat: 5g; Unsaturated fat: 8g.

82. Squirrel Sausage

Preparation time: 15 minutes   **Cooking time:** 10 minutes   **Servings:** 4

Ingredients:

- 1 pound ground squirrel meat
- 1 teaspoon salt
- 1/2 teaspoon black pepper
- 1 teaspoon sage
- 1/2 teaspoon thyme
- 1/4 teaspoon cayenne pepper (optional for a spicy kick)
- 2 tablespoon cold water

Directions:

1. In a large mixing bowl, combine the ground squirrel meat with salt, black pepper, sage, thyme, and cayenne pepper (if using). Mix well to ensure the spices are evenly distributed throughout the meat.

2. Gradually add the cold water to the squirrel mixture. This helps to keep the sausage moist during cooking. Mix until well combined.

3. Divide the mixture into equal portions and shape each portion into a sausage link or patty, depending on your preference.

4. Preheat your air fryer to 400°F (200°C). Once heated, place the squirrel sausages in the air fryer basket, ensuring they are not touching to allow for even cooking.

5. Cook for 10 minutes, turning the sausages halfway through the cooking time, until they are browned and cooked through.

6. Carefully remove the sausages from the air fryer and let them rest for a couple of minutes before serving.

Per serving: Calories: 160kcal; Carbs: 0g; Fiber: 0g; Sugars: 0g; Protein: 22g; Saturated fat: 2g; Unsaturated fat: 1g.

83. Heart Kebabs

Preparation time: 15 minutes   **Cooking time:** 15 minutes   **Servings:** 4

Ingredients:

- 1 pound beef or lamb heart, trimmed and cut into 1-inch cubes
- 2 tablespoons olive oil
- 1 teaspoon sea salt
- 1/2 teaspoon black pepper
- 1/2 teaspoon garlic powder
- 1/2 teaspoon smoked paprika
- Wooden or metal skewers

Directions:

1. Preheat your air fryer to 400°F (200°C). If using wooden skewers, soak them in water for at least 30 minutes to prevent burning.

2. In a large bowl, combine the heart cubes with olive oil, sea salt, black pepper, garlic powder, and smoked paprika. Toss until the meat is evenly coated with the seasonings.

3. Thread the heart cubes onto the skewers, leaving a small space between each piece to ensure even cooking.

4. Place the skewers in the air fryer basket, making sure they are not touching. You may need to cook in batches depending on the size of your air fryer.

5. Cook for 15 minutes, turning the skewers halfway through the cooking time, until the heart cubes are browned on the outside and reach your desired level of doneness.

6. Carefully remove the heart kebabs from the air fryer and let them rest for a few minutes before serving.

Per serving: Calories: 250kcal; Carbs: 0g; Fiber: 0g; Sugars: 0g; Protein: 34g; Saturated fat: 4g; Unsaturated fat: 5g.

84. Kidney Pie

Preparation time: 5 minutes   **Cooking time:** 25 minutes   **Servings:** 4

Ingredients:

- 1 pound beef kidneys, cleaned and diced
- 1 tablespoon olive oil
- 1 teaspoon salt
- 1/2 teaspoon black pepper
- 1/2 teaspoon thyme
- 2 cups ground pork rinds (for crust)
- 1 egg (for crust binding)
- 1/4 cup beef broth

Directions:

1. Preheat your air fryer to 375°F (190°C).
2. In a skillet over medium heat, heat the olive oil. Add the diced kidneys, salt, pepper, and thyme. Cook until the kidneys are browned on all sides, about 5 minutes.
3. In a bowl, mix the ground pork rinds with the egg to form a dough-like consistency. Press this mixture into the bottom and sides of a compatible air fryer pie dish to form a crust.
4. Spoon the cooked kidneys into the crust. Pour the beef broth over the kidneys. This will help keep the filling moist during cooking.
5. Place the pie dish in the air fryer basket. Cook for 20 minutes, or until the crust is golden and crispy.
6. Carefully remove the kidney pie from the air fryer and let it cool for a few minutes before serving.

Per serving: Calories: 320kcal; Carbs: 2g; Fiber: 0g; Sugars: 0g; Protein: 35g; Saturated fat: 8g; Unsaturated fat: 10g.

Meaty Bowls and Wraps Recipes

85. Beef Bowl

Preparation time: 10 minutes   **Cooking time:** 15 minutes   **Servings:** 2

Ingredients:

- 1 pound ground beef
- 1 teaspoon salt
- 1/2 teaspoon black pepper
- 1/2 teaspoon garlic powder

Directions:

1. Preheat your air fryer to 400°F (200°C).
2. In a medium bowl, season the ground beef with salt, black pepper, and garlic powder. Mix well to ensure the seasoning is evenly distributed.
3. Form the seasoned ground beef into small balls and flatten them into patties.
4. Place the beef patties in the air fryer basket, ensuring they are not touching to allow for even cooking.
5. Cook for 15 minutes, flipping the patties halfway through the cooking time, until they are browned on the outside and cooked through.
6. Once cooked, remove the beef patties from the air fryer and let them rest for a couple of minutes before breaking them into smaller pieces.
7. Divide the cooked beef into two bowls, creating a base for your beef bowl.

Per serving: Calories: 480kcal; Carbs: 0g; Fiber: 0g; Sugars: 0g; Protein: 44g; Saturated fat: 18g; Unsaturated fat: 20g.

86. Pork Wrap

Preparation time: 10 minutes   **Cooking time:** 15 minutes   **Servings:** 2

Ingredients:

- 1 pound pork tenderloin, sliced thinly
- 1 teaspoon salt
- 1/2 teaspoon black pepper
- 1 tablespoon olive oil
- 4 large lettuce leaves (for wrapping)
- Optional: Mustard or your favorite carnivore diet-approved sauce for serving

Directions:

1. Preheat your air fryer to 400°F (200°C).

2. Season the pork tenderloin slices evenly with salt and pepper.

3. Toss the seasoned pork slices with olive oil to ensure they are well-coated.

4. Place the pork slices in the air fryer basket in a single layer, ensuring they are not touching to allow for even cooking. You may need to cook in batches depending on the size of your air fryer.

5. Cook for 15 minutes, flipping the pork slices halfway through the cooking time, until they are fully cooked and have a slight crisp on the edges.

6. Once cooked, remove the pork slices from the air fryer and let them rest for a couple of minutes.

7. Place a few slices of pork on each lettuce leaf, add a dollop of mustard or your chosen sauce if desired, and wrap the lettuce around the pork to form a wrap.

8. Serve immediately and enjoy your delicious Pork Wrap.

Per serving: Calories: 300kcal; Carbs: 1g; Fiber: 0g; Sugars: 0g; Protein: 48g; Saturated fat: 3g; Unsaturated fat: 5g.

87. Chicken Caesar Wrap

Preparation time: 10 minutes   **Cooking time:** 15 minutes   **Servings:** 2

Ingredients:

- 2 chicken breasts (about 6 ounces each)
- Salt and pepper to taste
- 1 tablespoon olive oil
- 4 large lettuce leaves, preferably Romaine or iceberg for wrapping
- 2 tablespoons Caesar dressing (carnivore diet-approved, made with egg yolk, olive oil, anchovy, and seasoning)
- Optional: Shaved Parmesan cheese
- Optional: Anchovy fillets for additional flavor

Directions:

1. Season the chicken breasts with salt and pepper.

2. Heat the olive oil in a skillet over medium-high heat. Add the chicken breasts and cook for about 7-8 minutes on each side, or until fully cooked and golden brown. The internal temperature should reach 165°F (74°C).

3. Once cooked, remove the chicken from the skillet and let it rest for a few minutes before slicing into thin strips.

4. Lay out the lettuce leaves on a flat surface. Divide the sliced chicken equally and place it with the lettuce leaves.

5. Drizzle each with 1 tablespoon of Caesar dressing. If using, add shaved Parmesan cheese and anchovy fillets to taste.

6. Carefully roll each lettuce leaf to enclose the fillings, creating a wrap.

7. Serve immediately for the best texture and flavor.

Per serving: Calories: 290kcal; Carbs: 2g; Fiber: 1g; Sugars: 1g; Protein: 36g; Saturated fat: 3g; Unsaturated fat: 13ga.

88. Lamb Gyro Bowl

Preparation time: 10 minutes   **Cooking time:** 20 minutes   **Servings:** 2

Ingredients:

- 1 pound ground lamb
- 1 teaspoon salt
- 1/2 teaspoon black pepper
- 1/2 teaspoon garlic powder
- 1/2 teaspoon onion powder
- 1 tablespoon olive oil

Directions:

1. Preheat your air fryer to 400°F (200°C).
2. In a bowl, mix the ground lamb with salt, black pepper, garlic powder, and onion powder until well combined.
3. Form the lamb mixture into small patties or meatballs.
4. Brush each patty with olive oil to ensure a crispy exterior.
5. Place the lamb patties in the air fryer basket, making sure they are not touching to allow for even cooking.
6. Cook for 20 minutes, flipping halfway through the cooking time, until the lamb is fully cooked and has a crispy exterior.
7. Once cooked, remove the lamb from the air fryer and let it rest for a few minutes.
8. To assemble the gyro bowl, place the cooked lamb in a bowl. For those who include dairy in their carnivore diet, you may add a dollop of carnivore-friendly yogurt or sour cream on top, though this is optional.

Per serving: Calories: 480kcal; Carbs: 0g; Fiber: 0g; Sugars: 0g; Protein: 44g; Saturated fat: 20g; Unsaturated fat: 22g.

89. Duck Wrap

Preparation time: 10 minutes   **Cooking time:** 20 minutes   **Servings:** 2

Ingredients:

- 2 duck breasts
- 1 teaspoon salt
- 1/2 teaspoon black pepper
- 1 tablespoon olive oil
- 4 large lettuce leaves (for wrapping)
- Optional: Fresh herbs for garnish (such as thyme or rosemary)

Directions:

1. Preheat your air fryer to 360°F (182°C).
2. Season the duck breasts with salt and pepper.

3. Rub each breast with olive oil to ensure even cooking and a crispy finish.

4. Place the duck breasts in the air fryer basket and cook for 20 minutes, or until the internal temperature reaches 165°F (74°C) and the skin is crispy.

5. Once cooked, remove the duck breasts from the air fryer and let them rest for 5 minutes. This allows the juices to redistribute, ensuring the meat is moist and flavorful.

6. Thinly slice the duck breasts.

7. Place a portion of the sliced duck onto each lettuce leaf, wrap tightly, and garnish with fresh herbs if desired.

8. Serve immediately and enjoy the rich, satisfying flavors of your Duck Wrap.

Per serving: Calories: 310kcal; Carbs: 1g; Fiber: 0g; Sugars: 0g; Protein: 22g; Saturated fat: 5g; Unsaturated fat: 5g.

90. Venison Bowl

Preparation time: 10 minutes   **Cooking time:** 15 minutes   **Servings:** 2

Ingredients:

- 1 pound venison steak, cut into bite-sized pieces
- 1 tablespoon olive oil
- 1 teaspoon salt
- 1/2 teaspoon black pepper
- Optional: Fresh herbs (such as thyme or rosemary) for seasoning

Directions:

1. Preheat your air fryer to 400°F (200°C).

2. In a bowl, toss the venison pieces with olive oil, salt, pepper, and any optional herbs until well coated.

3. Arrange the venison pieces in the air fryer basket in a single layer, ensuring they are not touching to allow for even cooking.

4. Cook for 15 minutes, or until the venison is cooked through and slightly crispy on the outside.

5. Once cooked, carefully remove the venison from the air fryer and let it rest for a couple of minutes.

6. Serve the venison in bowls, either as is for a pure carnivore diet meal or with your choice of carnivore diet-approved sides.

Per serving: Calories: 320kcal; Carbs: 0g; Fiber: 0g; Sugars: 0g; Protein: 48g; Saturated fat: 3g; Unsaturated fat: 5g.

91. Bison Wrap

Preparation time: 10 minutes   **Cooking time:** 10 minutes   **Servings:** 2

Ingredients:

- 1/2 pound bison steak, thinly sliced
- 1 teaspoon salt
- 1/2 teaspoon black pepper
- 1 tablespoon olive oil
- 4 large lettuce leaves (such as romaine or iceberg) for wrapping

Directions:

1. Season the bison steak slices generously with salt and pepper.
2. Heat the olive oil in a skillet over medium-high heat. Add the bison slices and cook for about 2-3 minutes on each side, or until they reach your desired level of doneness.
3. Remove the bison from the skillet and let it rest for a couple of minutes. This allows the juices to redistribute, ensuring the meat is moist and flavorful.
4. Divide the cooked bison slices evenly among the lettuce leaves, placing them in the center of each leaf.
5. Carefully wrap the lettuce around the bison slices, tucking in the edges to secure the filling.
6. Serve immediately, enjoying the rich and tender flavors of the bison wrapped in the crisp, fresh lettuce.

Per serving: Calories: 220kcal; Carbs: 2g; Fiber: 1g; Sugars: 1g; Protein: 26g; Saturated fat: 3g; Unsaturated fat: 5g.

92. Turkey Lettuce Wrap

Preparation time: 10 minutes   **Cooking time:** 10 minutes   **Servings:** 4

Ingredients:

- 1 pound ground turkey
- 1 teaspoon salt
- 1/2 teaspoon black pepper
- 1 tablespoon olive oil
- 8 large lettuce leaves (preferably iceberg or butter lettuce for crunch)
- Optional: Hot sauce or mustard for serving

Directions:

1. Heat the olive oil in a skillet over medium heat. Add the ground turkey, salt, and pepper. Cook, stirring and breaking up the meat with a spatula, until the turkey is browned and cooked through, about 10 minutes.
2. While the turkey is cooking, rinse and pat dry the lettuce leaves, setting them aside for wrapping.
3. Once the turkey is fully cooked, remove the skillet from the heat and let it cool slightly.

4. To assemble the wraps, place a portion of the cooked turkey into the center of a lettuce leaf. If using, add a few drops of hot sauce or a smear of mustard on top of the turkey.

5. Fold the sides of the lettuce leaf in, then roll it up to enclose the filling. Repeat with the remaining lettuce leaves and turkey mixture.

6. Serve the turkey lettuce wraps immediately, with additional hot sauce or mustard on the side if desired.

Per serving: Calories: 180kcal; Carbs: 1g; Fiber: 0.5g; Sugars: 0g; Protein: 22g; Saturated fat: 2g; Unsaturated fat: 3g.

93. Elk Bowl

Preparation time: 10 minutes   **Cooking time:** 15 minutes   **Servings:** 2

Ingredients:

- 1 pound ground elk meat
- 1 teaspoon sea salt
- 1/2 teaspoon black pepper
- 1 tablespoon olive oil
- Optional: Fresh herbs (such as thyme or rosemary) for flavor

Directions:

1. Heat the olive oil in a skillet over medium-high heat. Add the ground elk meat, breaking it apart with a spoon.

2. Season the meat with sea salt and black pepper. If using, add fresh herbs for additional flavor.

3. Cook the elk meat for about 10-15 minutes, or until fully browned and cooked through, stirring occasionally to ensure even cooking.

4. Once the elk meat is ready, divide it into two bowls.

5. Serve hot, allowing the simple yet rich flavors of the elk to shine through. Optional: Garnish with additional fresh herbs for a burst of flavor and color.

Per serving: Calories: 320kcal; Carbs: 0g; Fiber: 0g; Sugars: 0g; Protein: 52g; Saturated fat: 5g; Unsaturated fat: 7g.

94. Rabbit Wrap

Preparation time: 10 minutes   **Cooking time:** 20 minutes   **Servings:** 2

Ingredients:

- 1 pound rabbit meat, cooked and shredded
- 2 large lettuce leaves (for wrapping)
- Salt and pepper to taste
- Optional: 1/2 teaspoon garlic powder

Directions:

1. Preheat your air fryer to 380°F (193°C).
2. Season the shredded rabbit meat with salt, pepper, and garlic powder (if using) to taste.
3. Place the seasoned rabbit meat in the air fryer basket, spreading it out for even cooking.
4. Cook for 10 minutes, or until the rabbit meat is crispy and heated through.
5. Carefully remove the rabbit meat from the air fryer and let it cool slightly.
6. Divide the cooked rabbit meat evenly among the lettuce leaves, placing it in the center of each leaf.
7. Roll the lettuce leaves tightly around the rabbit meat, securing with a toothpick if necessary.
8. Serve the rabbit wraps immediately, enjoying the crispy, juicy flavors of the rabbit meat encased in a fresh lettuce leaf.

Per serving: Calories: 220kcal; Carbs: 1g; Fiber: 0.5g; Sugars: 0g; Protein: 35g; Saturated fat: 1g; Unsaturated fat: 3g.

95. Pheasant Bowl

Preparation time: 10 minutes   **Cooking time:** 20 minutes   **Servings:** 2

Ingredients:

- 1 whole pheasant, breast meat removed and sliced
- 1 tablespoon olive oil
- Salt and pepper to taste
- Optional: Fresh herbs (such as thyme or rosemary) for seasoning

Directions:

1. Preheat your air fryer to 390°F (200°C).
2. Season the pheasant slices with salt, pepper, and optional herbs. Drizzle with olive oil to coat evenly.
3. Place the seasoned pheasant slices in the air fryer basket, ensuring they are spread out in a single layer for even cooking.
4. Cook for 20 minutes, flipping halfway through, until the pheasant is golden brown and cooked through.
5. Once done, remove the pheasant from the air fryer and let it rest for a few minutes.
6. Serve the pheasant slices in a bowl. For a complete carnivore diet-approved meal, consider pairing with a side of air-fried bacon or a dollop of animal fat mayo.

Per serving: Calories: 220kcal; Carbs: 0g; Fiber: 0g; Sugars: 0g; Protein: 35g; Saturated fat: 3g; Unsaturated fat: 5g.

96. Offal Taco Bowl

Preparation time: 10 minutes   **Cooking time:** 15 minutes   **Servings:** 2

Ingredients:

- 1/2 pound mixed offal (liver, heart, and kidney), finely chopped
- 1 tablespoon olive oil
- 1 teaspoon salt
- 1/2 teaspoon black pepper
- 1/2 teaspoon cumin
- 1/2 teaspoon smoked paprika
- 2 cups iceberg lettuce, shredded
- Optional: Fresh cilantro and lime wedges for garnish

Directions:

1. Preheat your air fryer to 400°F (200°C).
2. In a bowl, toss the chopped offal with olive oil, salt, black pepper, cumin, and smoked paprika until well coated.
3. Spread the seasoned offal in a single layer in the air fryer basket, ensuring the pieces are not touching for even cooking.
4. Cook for 15 minutes, stirring halfway through, until the offal is fully cooked and slightly crispy on the edges.
5. While the offal is cooking, prepare the taco bowls by dividing the shredded lettuce between two bowls.
6. Once the offal is cooked, evenly distribute it atop the shredded lettuce in each bowl.
7. Garnish with fresh cilantro and lime wedges if desired and serve immediately.

Per serving: Calories: 220kcal; Carbs: 2g; Fiber: 1g; Sugars: 0g; Protein: 20g; Saturated fat: 3g; Unsaturated fat: 5g.

Snacks and Sides Recipes

97. Pork Rind Nachos

Preparation time: 10 minutes   **Cooking time:** 15 minutes   **Servings:** 4

Ingredients:

- 4 cups pork rinds
- 1 pound ground beef
- 1 teaspoon salt
- 1/2 teaspoon black pepper
- 1 cup shredded cheddar cheese
- Optional: Jalapeños for topping

Directions:

1. Preheat your air fryer to 400°F (200°C).
2. In a skillet over medium heat, cook the ground beef with salt and pepper for 8-10 minutes, or until browned and fully cooked. Drain any excess fat.
3. Arrange the pork rinds in a single layer at the bottom of an air fryer-safe pan or foil.
4. Evenly distribute the cooked ground beef over the pork rinds.
5. Sprinkle the shredded cheddar cheese on top of the ground beef.
6. Place the pan in the air fryer and cook for 5 minutes, or until the cheese is fully melted and bubbly.
7. If using, add jalapeños on top for an extra kick.
8. Carefully remove the pan from the air fryer and let it cool for a minute before serving.

Per serving: Calories: 540kcal; Carbs: 0g; Fiber: 0g; Sugars: 0g; Protein: 38g; Saturated fat: 18g; Unsaturated fat: 20g.

98. Carnivore Muffins

Preparation time: 5 minutes   **Cooking time:** 20 minutes   **Servings:** 2

Ingredients:

- 2 teaspoon butter
- 1 1/2 cups mozzarella cheese shredded
- 2 large eggs

Directions:

1. Preheat the oven to 350 °F (175°C).
2. Combine cheese and eggs together in a large mixing bowl.
3. Divide the batter and fill each muffin space evenly.

4. Cook for 20 minutes, until tops are golden brown.

5. Run a knife around the edges to loosen each muffin.

6. Remove from the pan and cool for a minute before serving.

Per serving: Calories: 108kcal; Carbs: 0g; Fiber: 0g; Sugars: 0g; Protein: 10g; Saturated fat: 3g; Unsaturated fat: 5g.

99. Chicken Skin Chips

Preparation time: 5 minutes　　　**Cooking time:** 15 minutes　　　**Servings:** 4

Ingredients:

- Chicken skin from 4 chicken thighs
- 1 teaspoon salt
- 1/2 teaspoon black pepper

Directions:

1. Preheat your air fryer to 360°F (182°C).

2. Pat the chicken skin dry with paper towels to remove any excess moisture. This step is crucial for achieving maximum crispiness.

3. Season the chicken skin evenly with salt and pepper.

4. Place the chicken skin in the air fryer basket in a single layer, ensuring they are not overlapping to allow for even cooking.

5. Cook for 15 minutes, or until the chicken skin is golden brown and crispy. You may need to shake the basket halfway through the cooking time to ensure even crispiness.

6. Carefully remove the chicken skin chips from the air fryer and place them on a paper towel-lined plate to absorb any excess oil.

7. Serve immediately and enjoy the crunchy, savory flavors of your Chicken Skin Chips.

Per serving: Calories: 150kcal; Carbs: 0g; Fiber: 0g; Sugars: 0g; Protein: 14g; Saturated fat: 5g; Unsaturated fat: 3g.

100. Lamb Fat Bombs

Preparation time: 10 minutes　　　**Cooking time:** 0 minutes　　　**Servings:** 8
(Freeze time: 1 hour)

Ingredients:

- 1 cup rendered lamb fat, melted
- 1/2 teaspoon salt
- Optional: 1/4 teaspoon rosemary powder for added flavor

Directions:

1. In a mixing bowl, combine the melted lamb fat with salt and optional rosemary powder. Stir until well mixed.
2. Pour the mixture into silicone molds of your choice, filling each cavity about three-quarters full.
3. Place the molds in the freezer and freeze for at least 1 hour, or until the fat bombs are solid.
4. Once solid, pop the Lamb Fat Bombs out of the molds and store them in an airtight container in the refrigerator.
5. Enjoy a Lamb Fat Bomb as a quick snack or energy boost whenever needed.

Per serving: Calories: 115kcal; Carbs: 0g; Fiber: 0g; Sugars: 0g; Protein: 0g; Saturated fat: 11g; Unsaturated fat: 1g.

101. Duck Cracklings

Preparation time: 5 minutes   **Cooking time:** 15 minutes   **Servings:** 4

Ingredients:

- Duck skin, trimmed and cut into 2-inch pieces
- 1 teaspoon salt
- 1/2 teaspoon black pepper

Directions:

1. Preheat your air fryer to 400°F (200°C).
2. Pat the duck skin dry with paper towels to remove any excess moisture. This step is crucial for achieving maximum crispiness.
3. Season the duck skin pieces evenly with salt and pepper.
4. Place the seasoned duck skin in the air fryer basket in a single layer, ensuring they are not overlapping to allow for even cooking.
5. Cook for 15 minutes, or until the duck skin is golden brown and crispy. Shake the basket halfway through the cooking time to ensure even crispiness.
6. Carefully remove the duck cracklings from the air fryer and let them cool on a paper towel-lined plate to absorb any excess fat.
7. Serve the duck cracklings immediately for the best texture and flavor.

Per serving: Calories: 100kcal; Carbs: 0g; Fiber: 0g; Sugars: 0g; Protein: 9g; Saturated fat: 4g; Unsaturated fat: 5g.

102. Scotch Eggs

Preparation time: 5 minutes **Cooking time:** 25 minutes **Servings:** 4

Ingredients:

- 2 pounds ground beef or chicken sausage
- 2 tablespoons salt
- 12 large hard boiled eggs

Directions:

1. Preheat your air fryer to 350°F (175°C).
2. In a large bowl, combine the ground beef or chicken sausage with salt. Mix well using your hands.
3. Divide the meat mixture into 12 equal portions and shape them into meatballs.
4. Flatten each meatball to form a thin circle.
5. Place a boiled egg in the center of each meat circle and wrap the meat around the egg, ensuring there are no gaps or holes.
6. Arrange the wrapped eggs in the air fryer basket, leaving some space between each one.
7. Cook in the air fryer for 15 minutes at 350°F (175°C) until the top of the meatballs looks cooked.
8. Carefully flip the meatballs over and continue cooking for another 10 minutes.
9. Serve the Scotch eggs immediately for the best texture and flavor.

Per serving: Calories: 270kcal; Carbs: 0g; Fiber: 0g; Sugars: 0g; Protein: 19g; Saturated fat: 7g; Unsaturated fat: 13g.

103. Bison Bites

Preparation time: 10 minutes **Cooking time:** 15 minutes **Servings:** 4

Ingredients:

- 1 pound ground bison meat
- 1 teaspoon salt
- 1/2 teaspoon black pepper
- Optional: 1/2 teaspoon garlic powder

Directions:

1. In a large bowl, mix the ground bison meat with salt, black pepper, and garlic powder (if using) until well combined.
2. Form the mixture into small, bite-sized balls, about 1 inch in diameter.
3. Preheat your air fryer to 400°F (200°C).
4. Place the bison balls in the air fryer basket, ensuring they are not touching to allow for even cooking.

5. Cook for 15 minutes, or until the bison bites are fully cooked and have a crispy exterior.

6. Carefully remove the bison bites from the air fryer and let them rest for a couple of minutes before serving.

Per serving: Calories: 220kcal; Carbs: 0g; Fiber: 0g; Sugars: 0g; Protein: 26g; Saturated fat: 3g; Unsaturated fat: 5g.

104. Mozzarella-Stuffed Chicken Breasts

Preparation time: 10 minutes   **Cooking time:** 20 minutes   **Servings:** 2

Ingredients:

- 2 boneless, skinless chicken breasts
- 4 slices bacon
- Salt and pepper, to taste
- 2 ounces mozzarella, sliced

Directions:

1. Preheat the air fryer to 375°F.
2. Cut a pocket into each chicken breast.
3. Season the chicken breasts with salt and pepper.
4. Stuff each pocket with the mozzarella slices.
5. Wrap each chicken breast with 2 slices of bacon.
6. Place the mozzarella-stuffed chicken breasts in the air fryer basket.
7. Air fry for 18-20 minutes, or until the chicken is cooked through and the bacon is crispy.

Per serving: Calories: 490kcal; Carbs: 0g; Fiber: 0g; Sugars: 0g; Protein: 39g; Saturated fat: 25g; Unsaturated fat: 10g.

105. Salmon with Lemon Dill Butter

Preparation time: 10 minutes   **Cooking time:** 12 minutes   **Servings:** 2

Ingredients:

- 2 salmon fillets
- 2 tablespoons butter, melted
- 1 tablespoon fresh lemon juice
- 1 tablespoon chopped fresh dill (optional)
- Salt and pepper, to taste

Directions:

1. Preheat the air fryer to 375°F.
2. Season the salmon fillets using salt and pepper.

3. In your small bowl, mix together melted butter, lemon juice, and chopped dill (optional).

4. Brush the lemon dill butter mixture over the salmon fillets.

5. Place salmon fillets in your air fryer basket.

6. Air fry 10-12 minutes, or until the salmon is cooked through then flakes easily with a fork.

Per serving: Calories: 356kcal; Carbs: 0g; Fiber: 0g; Sugars: 0g; Protein: 33g; Saturated fat: 7g; Unsaturated fat: 18g.

106. Butter Scallops

Preparation time: 10 minutes   **Cooking time:** 8 minutes   **Servings:** 2

Ingredients:

- 1/2 pound large scallops
- 2 tablespoons unsalted butter, melted
- 1 teaspoon garlic powder
- 1 tablespoon chopped fresh parsley
- Salt and pepper to taste

Directions:

1. Pat dry the scallops using paper towels then season using salt and pepper.

2. In your small bowl, mix together melted butter, garlic powder, and chopped parsley.

3. Preheat air fryer to 400°F (200°C) for 3 minutes.

4. Bring the seasoned scallops in your air fryer basket.

5. Drizzle the garlic butter mixture over the scallops.

6. Air fry 8 minutes, depending on the size of the scallops, until they are opaque and slightly golden on the edges.

7. Serve hot.

Per serving: Calories: 199kcal; Carbs: 4g; Fiber: 0g; Sugars: 0g; Protein: 18g; Saturated fat: 7g; Unsaturated fat: 5g.

107. Pheasant Pâté

Preparation time: 7 minutes   **Cooking time:** 30 minutes   **Servings:** 4

Ingredients:

- 1 pound pheasant meat, cooked and shredded
- 1/2 cup unsalted butter, melted
- 1 teaspoon salt
- 1/2 teaspoon black pepper
- 1/4 teaspoon thyme
- 1/4 cup heavy cream
- 2 tablespoons brandy (optional)

Directions:

1. Preheat your air fryer to 350°F (175°C).
2. In a food processor, combine the cooked, shredded pheasant meat, melted butter, salt, black pepper, and thyme. Pulse until the mixture is well combined and starts to form a paste.
3. Gradually add the heavy cream to the food processor, continuing to pulse until the mixture becomes smooth and creamy. For an extra layer of flavor, add the brandy and blend well.
4. Transfer the pâté mixture into a suitable air fryer-safe dish. Smooth the top with a spatula.
5. Cook in the air fryer for 35 minutes, or until the pâté is firm to the touch and slightly golden on top.
6. Once cooked, remove the pâté from the air fryer and let it cool to room temperature. Then, refrigerate for at least 2 hours before serving to allow the flavors to meld and the pâté to set.
7. Serve chilled, accompanied by carnivore diet-friendly sides or simply enjoy it by itself.

Per serving: Calories: 410kcal; Carbs: 0g; Fiber: 0g; Sugars: 0g; Protein: 25g; Saturated fat: 25g; Unsaturated fat: 10g.

108. Liver Chips

Preparation time: 10 minutes   **Cooking time:** 8 minutes   **Servings:** 4

Ingredients:

- 1/2 pound beef liver, thinly sliced
- 1 tablespoon olive oil
- Salt, to taste

Directions:

1. Preheat your air fryer to 375°F (190°C).
2. Pat the beef liver slices dry with paper towels to remove any excess moisture. This step is crucial for achieving a crispy texture.
3. Cut the liver slices into thin, chip-sized pieces.
4. In a bowl, toss the liver pieces with olive oil and salt until evenly coated.
5. Arrange the liver pieces in a single layer in the air fryer basket, ensuring they are not overlapping. You may need to work in batches depending on the size of your air fryer.
6. Cook for 8 minutes, or until the liver chips are crispy and slightly curled at the edges.
7. Carefully remove the liver chips from the air fryer and let them cool on a wire rack for a few minutes to maintain their crispiness.
8. Serve immediately as a crunchy, protein-rich snack.

Per serving: Calories: 150kcal; Carbs: 1g; Fiber: 0g; Sugars: 0g; Protein: 20g; Saturated fat: 2g; Unsaturated fat: 3g.

Homemade Sauces, Dips and Seasonings

Recipes

109. Carnivore BBQ Sauce

Preparation time: 5 minutes   **Cooking time:** 10 minutes   **Servings:** 8

Ingredients:

- 1 cup beef broth
- 2 tablespoons apple cider vinegar
- 1 tablespoon rendered beef tallow
- 1 teaspoon salt
- 1/2 teaspoon black pepper
- Optional: 1/4 teaspoon smoked paprika for added smokiness

Directions:

1. In a small saucepan, combine the beef broth, apple cider vinegar, and rendered beef tallow. Stir well to mix.
2. Season the mixture with salt, black pepper, and smoked paprika (if using). Stir them to ensure they are well combined
3. Place the saucepan over medium heat and bring the mixture to a simmer. Let it cook for about 10 minutes, or until the sauce has reduced by about a third and thickened slightly.
4. Once the sauce has reached your desired consistency, remove it from the heat and let it cool slightly.
5. Serve the Carnivore BBQ Sauce warm over your favorite carnivore diet-approved meats, such as steaks, ribs, or burgers.

Per serving: Calories: 25kcal; Carbs: 0g; Fiber: 0g; Sugars: 0g; Protein: 0g; Saturated fat: 2g; Unsaturated fat: 1g.

110. Animal Fat Mayo

Preparation time: 5 minutes   **Cooking time:** 0 minutes   **Servings:** 8

Ingredients:

- 1 cup rendered animal fat (beef tallow, duck fat, or pork lard), melted and cooled to room temperature
- 1 egg yolk, at room temperature
- 1 tablespoon lemon juice or vinegar
- Salt, to taste

Directions:

1. In a blender or food processor, combine the egg yolk, lemon juice or vinegar, and a pinch of salt. Blend these ingredients together until well mixed.

2. With the blender or food processor running on low speed, slowly drizzle in the rendered animal fat until the mixture begins to thicken and emulsify. This process should take about 1-2 minutes.

3. Once the mixture has reached a mayonnaise-like consistency, taste and adjust the seasoning with additional salt if necessary.

4. Transfer the animal fat mayo to a jar or an airtight container and refrigerate. Allow it to chill for at least 1 hour before serving to let the flavors meld and the mayo to set.

5. Serve your Animal Fat Mayo with your favorite carnivore diet dishes, using it as a dip, spread, or base for sauces.

Per serving: Calories: 255kcal; Carbs: 0g; Fiber: 0g; Sugars: 0g; Protein: 0.5g; Saturated fat: 25g; Unsaturated fat: 10g.

111. Bone Marrow Spread

Preparation time: 10 minutes   **Cooking time:** 15 minutes   **Servings:** 4

Ingredients:

- 4 beef marrow bones, cut into 2-inch pieces
- 1 teaspoon sea salt
- 1/2 teaspoon black pepper
- Optional: Fresh herbs (such as thyme or rosemary) for garnish

Directions:

1. Preheat your air fryer to 400°F (200°C).

2. Season the marrow bones with sea salt and black pepper.

3. Place the bones in the air fryer basket, marrow side up, ensuring they are not touching for even cooking.

4. Cook for 15 minutes, or until the marrow is soft and slightly bubbly.

5. Carefully remove the marrow bones from the air fryer. Using a small spoon, scoop out the marrow and place it in a mixing bowl.

6. Mash the marrow with a fork until it reaches a spreadable consistency. If desired, mix in fresh herbs for added flavor.

7. Serve the bone marrow spread immediately on carnivore diet-approved crackers or slices of meat, or store in an airtight container in the refrigerator for up to one week.

Per serving: Calories: 110kcal; Carbs: 0g; Fiber: 0g; Sugars: 0g; Protein: 7g; Saturated fat: 10g; Unsaturated fat: 3g.

112. Beef Tallow Butter

Preparation time: 5 minutes   **Cooking time:** 0 minutes   **Servings:** 8

Ingredients:

- 1 cup beef tallow, softened
- 1/2 teaspoon salt
- Optional: 1/4 teaspoon garlic powder for added flavor

Directions:

1. In a medium mixing bowl, combine the softened beef tallow with salt, and if desired, garlic powder. Mix well until the ingredients are fully incorporated.
2. Using an electric mixer, whip the mixture on high speed for 3 to 4 minutes, or until it becomes light and fluffy, resembling the consistency of traditional butter.
3. Transfer the whipped Beef Tallow Butter to a serving dish or container. If not serving immediately, cover and store in the refrigerator.
4. Allow the Beef Tallow Butter to soften slightly at room temperature for a few minutes before serving for easy spreading.

Per serving: Calories: 115kcal; Carbs: 0g; Fiber: 0g; Sugars: 0g; Protein: 0g; Saturated fat: 12g; Unsaturated fat: 3g.

113. Duck Fat Aioli

Preparation time: 5 minutes   **Cooking time:** 0 minutes   **Servings:** 8

Ingredients:

- 1/2 cup duck fat, melted and cooled
- 2 egg yolks
- 1 tablespoon lemon juice
- 1 teaspoon Dijon mustard
- 1 garlic clove, minced
- Salt and pepper to taste

Directions:

1. In a food processor, combine the egg yolks, lemon juice, Dijon mustard, and minced garlic. Pulse until the mixture is well blended.
2. With the food processor running on low, slowly drizzle in the melted duck fat until the mixture thickens and emulsifies, forming a smooth aioli.
3. Season the aioli with salt and black pepper to taste. Pulse a few more times to incorporate the seasonings.
4. Transfer the aioli to a serving bowl or storage container. If not serving immediately, cover and refrigerate until needed. The aioli will thicken further as it chills.

5. Serve the Duck Fat Aioli as a dip, spread, or condiment with your favorite carnivore diet-approved dishes.

Per serving: Calories: 122kcal; Carbs: 0g; Fiber: 0g; Sugars: 0g; Protein: 1g; Saturated fat: 4g; Unsaturated fat: 8g.

114. Pork Lard Salsa

Preparation time: 5 minutes   **Cooking time:** 0 minutes   **Servings:** 4

Ingredients:

- 1/2 cup rendered pork lard, melted
- 1 tablespoon apple cider vinegar
- 1 teaspoon salt
- 1/2 teaspoon ground black pepper
- 1/2 teaspoon chili powder
- 1/2 teaspoon garlic powder
- 1/2 teaspoon onion powder

Directions:

1. In a mixing bowl, combine the melted pork lard with apple cider vinegar, salt, ground black pepper, chili powder, garlic powder, and onion powder. Whisk together until well blended.
2. Taste the salsa and adjust the seasoning if necessary, according to your preference.
3. Let the salsa sit for a few minutes to allow the flavors to meld together.
4. Serve the Pork Lard Salsa alongside your favorite carnivore diet dishes, such as grilled steaks, roasted chicken, or air-fried fish, for an added burst of flavor.

Per serving: Calories: 115kcal; Carbs: 0g; Fiber: 0g; Sugars: 0g; Protein: 0g; Saturated fat: 10g; Unsaturated fat: 3g.

115. Bison Bone Broth

Preparation time: 10 minutes   **Cooking time:** 24 hours   **Servings:** 8

Ingredients:

- 4 pounds of bison bones (a mix of marrow bones and bones with a bit of meat on them)
- 2 tablespoons apple cider vinegar
- 1 gallon of water
- Salt, to taste
- Optional: 1 onion, 2 carrots, and 2 celery stalks for added flavor

Directions:

1. If using, roughly chop the onion, carrots, and celery. No need to peel them, as the broth will be strained.
2. Place the bison bones in a large stockpot or slow cooker. Add the chopped vegetables if using.

3. Pour in the apple cider vinegar and water, ensuring the bones and vegetables are fully submerged.

4. Bring the mixture to a boil over high heat, then reduce the heat to low, allowing it to simmer gently. For the richest flavor and maximum nutrient extraction, simmer for 24 hours. Skim off any foam or impurities that rise to the surface during the first few hours of cooking.

5. After 24 hours, remove the pot from the heat. Let the broth cool slightly before straining it through a fine-mesh sieve to remove the bones and any solid bits.

6. Season the broth with salt to taste. For a clearer broth, you can further strain it through cheesecloth.

7. Serve the broth warm, or let it cool completely before storing it in the refrigerator or freezer. The broth will keep in the refrigerator for up to 5 days or can be frozen for up to 3 months.

Per serving: Calories: 50kcal; Carbs: 0g; Fiber: 0g; Sugars: 0g; Protein: 6g; Saturated fat: 0g; Unsaturated fat: 0g.

116. Chicken Liver Pâté

Preparation time: 10 minutes   **Cooking time:** 15 minutes   **Servings:** 4

Ingredients:

- 1 pound chicken livers, cleaned and trimmed
- 2 tablespoons unsalted butter
- 1/4 cup heavy cream
- 1 small onion, finely chopped
- 2 cloves garlic, minced

- 1 teaspoon fresh thyme leaves (optional)
- 1/2 teaspoon salt
- 1/4 teaspoon black pepper
- 2 tablespoons brandy or cognac (optional)

Directions:

1. Preheat your air fryer to 370°F.

2. In a skillet over medium heat, melt 1 tablespoon of butter. Add the onion and garlic, sautéing until translucent, about 3-4 minutes.

3. Add the chicken livers to the skillet, cooking until they are browned on the outside but still slightly pink in the middle, approximately 5 minutes.

4. Stir in the thyme, salt, pepper, and brandy (if using), cooking for an additional 2 minutes.

5. Transfer the liver mixture to a food processor, adding the remaining butter and heavy cream. Blend until the mixture is smooth.

6. Spoon the pâté into a serving dish or individual ramekins. For best flavor, cover and refrigerate for at least 2 hours before serving.

7. Serve chilled. The pâté can be stored in the refrigerator for up to 5 days.

Per serving: Calories: 292kcal; Carbs: 4g; Fiber: 0g; Sugars: 1g; Protein: 19g; Saturated fat: 10g; Unsaturated fat: 5g.

117. Fish Roe Dip

Preparation time: 5 minutes   **Cooking time:** 0 minutes   **Servings:** 4
(Freeze time: 30 minutes)

Ingredients:

- 1 cup fish roe (such as salmon or trout roe)
- 1/2 cup sour cream
- 1 tablespoon lemon juice
- Salt, to taste

Directions:

1. In a mixing bowl, gently combine the fish roe with sour cream and lemon juice until well mixed. Be careful not to break the roe sacs to maintain their texture.
2. Season the dip with a pinch of salt, adjusting to your taste.
3. Refrigerate the dip for at least 30 minutes before serving to allow the flavors to meld together.
4. Serve chilled, accompanied by carnivore diet-approved sides or simply enjoy it by itself for a pure taste experience.

Per serving: Calories: 98kcal; Carbs: 1g; Fiber: 0g; Sugars: 1g; Protein: 6g; Saturated fat: 3g; Unsaturated fat: 2g.

118. Venison Gravy

Preparation time: 5 minutes   **Cooking time:** 15 minutes   **Servings:** 4

Ingredients:

- 1 cup venison stock
- Drippings from cooked venison
- 1 tablespoon butter
- 1 tablespoon almond flour
- Salt and pepper, to taste

Directions:

1. In a saucepan over medium heat, melt the butter.
2. Stir in the almond flour, whisking continuously to form a smooth paste or roux. Cook for 2 minutes until the mixture turns slightly golden.
3. Gradually add the venison stock to the roux, continuing to whisk to prevent any lumps from forming.
4. Bring the mixture to a simmer, adding the drippings from the cooked venison. Allow the gravy to simmer for 10 minutes, or until it thickens to your desired consistency.
5. Season with salt and pepper to taste.
6. Once the gravy has reached the perfect thickness, remove it from the heat and let it sit for a minute before serving.
7. Serve the venison gravy hot, alongside your favorite carnivore diet dishes.

Per serving: Calories: 70kcal; Carbs: 1g; Fiber: 0g; Sugars: 0g; Protein: 4g; Saturated fat: 3g; Unsaturated fat: 2g.

119. Garlic Butter Dip

Preparation time: 5 minutes   **Cooking time:** 15 minutes   **Servings:** 4

Ingredients:

- 4 tablespoons unsalted butter, melted
- 2 cloves garlic, minced
- 1 tablespoon chopped fresh parsley
- Salt to taste

Directions:

1. In a mixing bowl, gently combine the butter with garlic and parsley until well mixed.
2. Season the dip with a pinch of salt, adjusting to your taste.
3. Refrigerate the dip for at least 30 minutes before serving to allow the flavors to meld together.
4. Serve chilled, accompanied by meat meal, or simply enjoy it by itself for a pure taste experience.

Per serving: Calories: 400kcal; Carbs: 0g; Fiber: 0g; Sugars: 0g; Protein: 1g; Saturated fat: 24g; Unsaturated fat: 16g.

120. Turkey Fat Dressing

Preparation time: 5 minutes   **Cooking time:** 0 minutes   **Servings:** 4

Ingredients:

- 1/2 cup rendered turkey fat, melted
- 1 teaspoon salt
- 1/2 teaspoon black pepper
- Optional: 1/4 teaspoon garlic powder for added flavor

Directions:

1. In a small mixing bowl, whisk together the melted turkey fat, salt, black pepper, and garlic powder (if using) until well combined.
2. Let the dressing cool slightly to thicken, about 5 minutes, stirring occasionally to maintain a smooth consistency.
3. Once thickened to your liking, taste and adjust the seasoning if necessary.
5. Serve the Turkey Fat Dressing immediately over your chosen dish, or store in an airtight container in the refrigerator for up to one week. Gently reheat before serving if the fat solidifies.

Per serving: Calories: 115kcal; Carbs: 0g; Fiber: 0g; Sugars: 0g; Protein: 0g; Saturated fat: 3g; Unsaturated fat: 8g.

Shopping List

Embark on your carnivore diet journey with confidence using my comprehensive shopping list. Designed to streamline your grocery shopping experience, this carefully curated guide ensures you have everything you need to create flavorful and satisfying meals. From premium cuts of meat to essential seasonings and spices, each item has been thoughtfully selected to support your carnivorous lifestyle. Whether you're a seasoned carnivore or new to the diet, my shopping list empowers you to make informed choices and embark on a delicious journey towards your health and wellness goals. Say goodbye to confusion in the aisles and hello to a hassle-free shopping experience tailored to your dietary needs.

Meat

- Bacon
- Bear steaks
- Beef kidneys
- Beef liver
- Beef ribs
- Beef sirloin
- Beef tenderloin
- Bison ribs
- Chorizo sausage
- Filet Mignon steaks
- Ground bison meat
- Ground elk meat
- Ground lamb
- Ground moose meat
- Ground pork
- Ground squirrel meat
- Ground venison
- Ham steaks
- Lamb hearts
- Lamb kidneys
- Lamb liver
- Lamb ribs
- Lamb shoulder
- Lamb steaks
- Lean beef

- Pork belly
- Pork chops
- Pork loin roast
- Pork spare ribs
- Rack of lamb
- T-Bone steaks
- Venison steaks

Poultry

- Chicken breasts
- Chicken livers
- Chicken sausage
- Chicken skin
- Chicken thighs
- Chicken wings
- Duck breasts
- Duck skin
- Ground turkey
- Turkey bacon

Fish and Seafood

- Cod fillets
- Crab legs
- Fish roe
- Halibut fillets

- Lobster tails
- Mackerel
- Oysters
- Salmon fillets
- Sardines
- Scallops
- Shrimp
- Swordfish steaks
- Tuna steaks

Egg

- Eggs

Dairy

- Cheddar cheese
- Heavy cream
- Mozzarella cheese
- Parmesan cheese
- Sour cream

Fats and Oils

- Beef tallow
- Duck fat
- Olive oil
- Pork lard

- Sesame oil

Herbs and Spices

- Black pepper
- Cayenne pepper
- Chili powder
- Chives
- Cilantro
- Cumin
- Dried oregano
- Dried rosemary
- Dried sage
- Dried thyme
- Garlic
- Ginger
- Nutmeg
- Onion
- Paprika
- Parsley
- Salt

Miscellaneous

- Almond flour
- Apple cider vinegar
- Beef broth
- Beef stock
- Brandy or cognac
- Caesar dressing
- Chicken broth
- Chicken stock
- Fish stock
- Honey
- Lemon
- Pork stock
- Soy sauce
- Turkey stock
- Venison stock

30-Day Meal Plan

Day	Breakfast	Lunch	Dinner	Snack
1	Air-Fried Bacon Strips	Pork Belly Bites	Pork Wrap	Pork Rind Nachos
2	Sausage Patties	Pork Loin Roast	Lamb Chops	Carnivore Muffins
3	Egg Muffins	Chorizo Bites	Chicken Caesar Wrap	Chicken Skin Chips
4	Pork Belly Crisp	Spare Ribs	Bison Burger	Lamb Fat Bombs
5	Steak & Eggs	Ham Steaks	Duck Wrap	Duck Cracklings
6	Turkey Bacon Crisp	Bacon and Egg Bites	T-Bone Steak	Scotch Eggs
7	Duck Breast	Chicken Thighs	Bison Wrap	Bison Bites
8	Venison Sausage	Turkey Meatballs	Rack of Lamb	Mozzarella-Stuffed Chicken Breasts
9	Chicken Liver Pâté	Spices-Stuffed Chicken	Turkey Lettuce Wrap	Salmon with Lemon Dill Butter
10	Lamb Chops	Chicken Wings	Ground Lamb	Butter Scallops
11	Bison Burger	Turkey Breast	Elk Burgers	Pheasant Pâté
12	Chicken Liver Pâté	Roasted Chicken	Rabbit Wrap	Liver Chips
13	Venison Sausage	Lamb Gyro Bowl	Lamb Steaks	Chicken Skin Chips
14	Salmon Fillets	Duck Wrap	Bear Steak	Scotch Eggs
15	Steak & Eggs	Cod Fillets	Duck Liver	Duck Cracklings
16	Bison Burger	Italian Herb Crusted Beef Tenderloin	Spiced Lamb Chops	Bison Bites
17	Air-Fried Bacon Strips	Venison Bowl	Pheasant Bowl	Lamb Fat Bombs
18	Sausage Patties	Elk Burgers	Elk Bowl	Pheasant Pâté
19	Egg Muffins	Lamb Gyro Bowl	Lamb Liver	Liver Chips
20	Pork Belly Bites	Chicken Wings	Bison Ribs	Duck Cracklings
21	Turkey Bacon Crisp	Chicken Liver	Lamb Burgers	Scotch Eggs
22	Duck Breast	Chicken Drumsticks	Lamb Ribs	Chicken Skin Chips
23	Venison Sausage	T-Bone Steak	Bison Burger	Bison Bites

24	Chicken Liver Pâté	Lamb Shoulder	Lamb Steaks	Butter Scallops
25	Air-Fried Bacon Strips	Turkey Meatballs	Rack of Lamb	Salmon with Lemon Dill Butter
26	Lamb Chops	Chicken Thighs	Ground Lamb	Mozzarella-Stuffed Chicken Breasts
27	Bison Burger	Turkey Breast	Lamb Burgers	Pheasant Pâté
28	Turkey Bacon Crisp	Roasted Chicken	Lamb Steaks	Liver Chips
29	Egg Muffins	Lamb Gyro Bowl	Elk Burgers	Chicken Skin Chips
30	Salmon Fillets	Crab Legs	Bear Steak	Scotch Eggs

Conversion Chart

Volume Equivalents (Liquid)

US Standard	US Standard (ounces)	Metric (approximate)
2 tablespoons	1 fl. oz.	30 mL
¼ cup	2 fl. oz.	60 mL
½ cup	4 fl. oz.	120 mL
1 cup	8 fl. oz.	240 mL
1½ cups	12 fl. oz.	355 mL
2 cups or 1 pint	16 fl. oz.	475 mL
4 cups or 1 quart	32 fl. oz.	1 L
1 gallon	128 fl. oz.	4 L

Volume Equivalents (Dry)

US Standard	Metric (approximate)
⅛ teaspoon	0.5 mL
¼ teaspoon	1 mL
½ teaspoon	2 mL
¾ teaspoon	4 mL
1 teaspoon	5 mL
1 tablespoon	15 mL
¼ cup	59 mL
⅓ cup	79 mL
½ cup	118 mL
⅔ cup	156 mL
¾ cup	177 mL
1 cup	235 mL
2 cups or 1 pint	475 mL
3 cups	700 mL
4 cups or 1 quart	1 L

Air Fryer Temperatures

Fahrenheit (F)	Celsius (C) (approximate)
175°F	79°C
200°F	93°C
225°F	107°C
250°F	121°C
275°F	135°C
300°F	149°C
325°F	163°C
350°F	177°C
375°F	191°C
400°F	204°C
425°F	218°C
450°F	232°C
475°F	246°C

Weight Equivalents

US Standard	Metric (approximate)
1 tablespoon	15 g
½ ounce	15 g
1 ounce	30 g
2 ounces	60 g
4 ounces	115 g
8 ounces	225 g
12 ounces	340 g
16 ounces or 1 pound	455 g

Conclusion

As we wrap up this journey through the Carnivore Diet Air Fryer Cookbook for Beginners, it's essential to reflect on the transformative path you've embarked upon. Embracing the carnivore diet with the innovative use of an air fryer has opened up a new world of culinary possibilities, designed to fit seamlessly into your active and health-conscious lifestyle. This guide has not only introduced you to the fundamentals of the carnivore diet and the efficiency of air frying but has also equipped you with a diverse collection of recipes to ensure your meals remain enjoyable, nutritious, and straightforward to prepare.

The transition to a carnivore diet, supported by the convenience of air frying, represents a significant step towards achieving your health and wellness goals, including weight loss and increased energy levels. By focusing on high-quality, nutrient-dense animal products, you've learned to nourish your body in a way that aligns with its natural needs, all while enjoying the simplicity and quickness of meal preparation that air frying offers.

Remember, the key to sustained success with the carnivore diet lies in the quality of the ingredients you choose and the consistency with which you apply the principles outlined in this cookbook. Opting for grass-fed, organic, and wild-caught options whenever possible will enhance the nutritional benefits of your meals, supporting your health journey even further.

As you continue to explore and experiment with the recipes provided, feel encouraged to adjust and tailor them to your taste preferences and nutritional requirements. The carnivore diet is highly personalizable, and with the air fryer as your culinary companion, you have the flexibility to create meals that are not only healthy and quick to prepare but also deeply satisfying.

Your adventure doesn't end here. The world of carnivore diet cooking is vast and ever evolving, and your air fryer is a tool that unlocks endless possibilities for innovation in the kitchen. Continue to engage with the carnivore diet community, share your discoveries, and seek inspiration from fellow carnivores who are also on this path to wellness.

In embracing the carnivore diet and mastering the art of air frying, you've taken control of your health and well-being in a way that is both empowering and delicious. Here's to many more days of vibrant health, energy, and mouthwatering meals prepared in your air fryer.

Recipe Index

Pork Wrap; 70
Quail; 35
Quail Eggs; 65
Rabbit Wrap; 75
Rack of Lamb; 47
Ribeye Steak; 40
Roasted Chicken; 37
Salmon Fillets; 20
Salmon Steaks; 55
Salmon with Lemon Dill Butter; 82
Sausage Links; 29
Sausage Patties; 16
Scotch Eggs; 81
Sesame Beef Skewers; 43
Sirloin Tips; 44
Spare Ribs; 26

Spiced Lamb Chops; 53
Spices-Stuffed Chicken; 33
Squirrel Sausage; 67
Steak & Eggs; 18
T-Bone Steak; 43
Tuna Steaks; 55
Turkey Bacon Crisp; 21
Turkey Breast; 34
Turkey Fat Dressing; 91
Turkey Lettuce Wrap; 74
Turkey Meatballs; 32
Venison Bowl; 73
Venison Gravy; 90
Venison Sausage; 22
Venison Steak; 62

Air Fryer Series

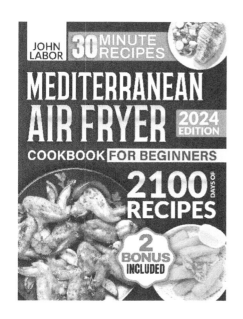 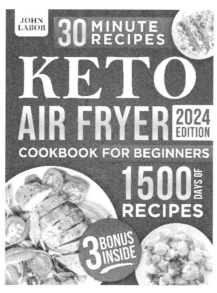 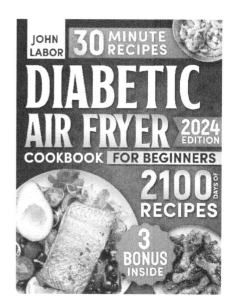

AVAILABLE ON AMAZON!

Hobbies and Free Time Series

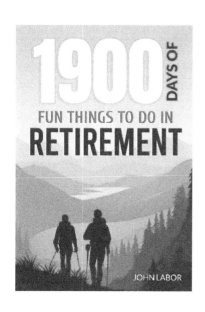 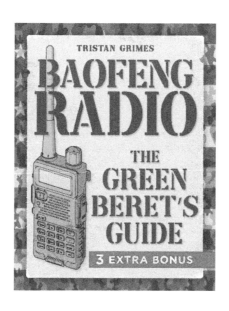 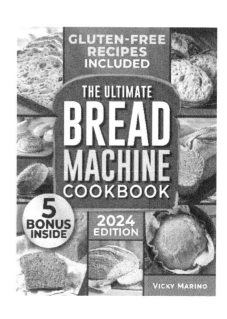

Made in the USA
Las Vegas, NV
19 October 2024